FIRST EDITION

THE ENCYCLOPEDIA
OF
HOMOEOPATHIC
FORMULAS

CLINIC AND FAMILY TREATMENT GUIDE

1400 Formulas for Diseases & Symptoms

(The Quick Remedy Finder)

By

DR. MAJOR (R)

Saif-ud-Din Saif

MBBS, MPH, RMP, RHMP

(All rights of publication and translation of this book are reserved with the writer)

Author: *Maj (Retd)*
DR. Professor
SAIF-UD-DIN SAIF
M.B; B.S, M.P.H, RMP, RHMP

The author is Professor of Community Medicine. He is qualified in the fields of Allopathic, Homoeopathic and Radiesthesia / Radionics systems of medicine. He has 24 years of teaching experience at M.B; B.S and post graduate level in various universities of Pakistan.

Cell Phone / Whatsapp: +92321-5827435
Email: drsaif1919@gmail.com

Other Books of Author:

1. Pharmacology: Classification and Doses (allopathy)
2. Rahnuma-e-Homeopath (Urdu)
3. Allergy-Allopathic and Homoeopathic Treatment (Urdu)
4. Research papers and articles on various topics

Table of Contents

1. Preface-Acknowledgment............................... 1
2. Introduction to Homeopathy......................... 4
   a. Definition... 4
   b. Introduction of Homeopathy..................... 4
   c. Aim of Homeopathy................................ 4
   d. The Founder of Homeopathy.................... 5
   e. The Vitalistic Principle and Higher Purpose of Existence... 5
   f. The Provings of Remedies........................ 6
   g. How Does it Work?................................. 7
   h. Mechanism of Action of Homeopathic Remedies... 8
   i. What is so Special about Homeopathy............ 9
   j. Selection of Remedy................................ 11
   k. Selection of Potency................................ 11
3. How to use this book (Instructions for Doctors)................................ 13
4. Final Book - A to Z Diseases, Symptoms, Organs, Formulas with potencies.. 17
5. Abbreviation table.. 196
6. Alphabetic index of diseases and symptoms........ 203

PREFACE

In the name of Allah, the most Beneficent the most Merciful

Praise be to ALLAH, the Lord of the Universe, and greetings and blessings on MUHEMMED, the Last of the Prophets, as well as his household and Companions.

Finding the *simillimum* (the exactly similar remedy to the totality of the patient) is the ideal approach according to classical Homoeopathy but it needs thorough knowledge of materia medica, philosophy, experience and lot of time for every patient which is not possible in present days. That's why successful classical Hahnemanian homoepaths are very few.

One of the Hahnemanns close associates named Ageidie, the personal physician to the prince of Prussia informed Hahnemann of his experiences of using multiple, mixed homoeopathic remedies to cure illnesses. Ageidie's results impressed Hahnemann, who then reported them at a seminar of homoeopathic physicians and suggested experimenting with such mixed remedies.

It has been observed that the complicated cases do not respond well or at all to the single remedy, probably due to wrong selection of remedy or due to the pollution of air, water and food with trace quantities of toxic substances, cigarette smoking and passive smoking. Tobacco chewing, drug ingestion, background radiation, chlorination and pollution of drinking water, adulteration of food and preservatives; other chemicals in food and beverages also antidote the effects of homoeopathic remedies. It necessitates the use of complementary remedies to neutralise the effects of such pollutants.

The famous dictum of Hahnemann is

"Experiment and see the results and hold fast to what is proved".

The same dictum inspired me to devise and prove the efficacy of the mixed remedies and present the research work to the profession. This will indeed help the practitioners in treating the patients in a much better, speedy and convenient way. It will also contribute to the cause of the profession. That's the sole aim behind this venture. These formulas have following advantages.

1. Immediate curative and palliative response have been observed. Thus, it saves the time and satisfies the patients and the doctor.

2. Results are better and permanent.

3. No aggravation or healing crisis occurs, which is more common with the single remedy (high potency) treatment.

4. Complicated cases respond better to formulas than a single remedy. Thus, formulas have a wider and deeper spectrum of action than a single remedy.

5. Most of the formulas in this book has been carefully and repeatedly tested by me.

6. In many cases remedies behave better in a formula than they act when applied alone.

7. No toxic side effects have been observed in the potency range specified in this work.

8. By repeated usage of formulas and with experience, one can attain the expertise to select the simillimum or single remedy out of a well selected formula. It is therefore a journey from formula to the art of classical single remedy selection.

I wish to express my appreciation and gratitude to Dr. Tanvir Ahmed, Dr. Sohail Akhtar Malik, Dr. Liaqat Ali Shahzad, Syed Ishtiaq Hussain Shah, Mr. Zahid Hussain and all others for their valuable work towards the compilation of this book. Suggestions from readers are most welcome for further improvement.

I present this work to the profession with a pride, confidence and hope that readers will use these formulas in their clinical practice and have results better than ever before *(Insha-Allah)*.

Rawalpindi, Pakistan **Dr. Major (R)**
May 19th 2020 **SAIF-UD DIN SAIF**

HOMOEOPATHY

Definition

"A rational system (science & art) of healing based on the principles that agents which produce certain signs and symptoms in healthy individuals, also cures these signs and symptoms in the sick and that the more a drug is diluted, the more powerful it becomes."

Introduction

The principle of *"law of similars"* or *"like curing like"* is about 200 years old. Although it has been opposed by the medical profession but modern medical men are not aware of the fact that they themselves are using the same principle in everyday medical practice. For example, the modern immunization system or vaccination against poliomyelitis, cholera, typhoid fever, diphtheria, hepatitis and other infectious diseases are being done on the "*like cures like principle*". Through these vaccines a micro dose of dead or altered bacteria or viruses is introduced into the body so that body could build up its own defences against those particular organisms. In this system it is claimed that antigenicity (antibody producing capacity) of pathogenic organisms is retained but their toxicity is reduced. Other examples are the usage of pollen to desensitize the patients; the use of x-rays and radium known to cause cancer, is being used to cure cancer.

The rational behind the principle is that a substance that actually induces exactly similar symptoms to the disease is probably stimulating the disease-fighting systems in the body and so curing the condition.

AIM OF HOMEOPATHY

To cure gently, rapidly, certainly and permanently without any toxic side effects; choosing in every case of disease, a medicine which can itself produce an artificial disease similar to the disorder to be treated. The artificial disease should be exactly similar but more severe than the actual disease. It has to be

THE FOUNDER OF HOMOEOPATHY

The celebrated German physician *Christian Samuel Freidrich Hahnemann* was born on 10th April 1755 in *Meissen*, Prussia (now in East Germany). He discovered Homoeopathy in 1790, two centuries ago. He graduated in Medicine in 1779 at Erlangen. In 1796 he published a booklet on *"like cures like"*. In 1810 he published the first edition of *"**Rational Healing (the Organon of Healing Art)**"* which presented the principles of homoeopathic doctrine. He published its five editions and the sixth was published after his death, in twentieth century. In 1811 & 1812 his Materia Medica was published in six volumes. In 1828 he published *"**Chronic Diseases**"*. He died in 1843 at the age of 88 years and was burried in a small cemetry in Monmartre. He was reburried in Pire Lachese in 1898, in the company of the immortals of France, and his tomb finally permitted to bear the inscription he had requested; ***Non inutilis vixi****("I have not lived in vain")*. He was real genius. A linguist, who was expert in sixteen languages, a master of chemistry and a Doctor of Medicine. Since 1790 to 1842 Hahnemann kept on testing (proving) the medicinal substances on himself, his friends and his pupils, in order to determine their physical, mental and moral effects precisely. He tested about one hundred agents upon himself. It is quite interesting that the provings had never been detrimental to health, but on the contrary, they raised the resistance of the provers.

"THE VITALISTIC PRINCIPLE AND HIGHER PURPOSES OF OUR EXISTENCE"

"In the healthy condition of man, the spiritual vital force (autocracy), the dynamis that animates the material body (organism), rules with unbounded sway, and retains all parts of the organism in admirable, harmonious, vital operations, as regards both sensations and function, so that our indwelling, reason-gifted mind can freely employ this living, healthy instrument for the higher purposes of our existence."

(Aphorism.9 "The Organon of Medicine" S. Hahnemann)

THE PROVINGS?

Homoeopathic proving was aimed at eliciting the detailed and precise physical, mental and moral sings and symptoms, alongwith the subjective sensations. The precise nature and modalities of all the symptoms, especially the emotional ones can only be obtained from human beings. Examples of such psychological and emotional symptoms are as under, alongwith their treatment.

Depression to the verge of suicide	Aurum metallicum
The insane jealousy of	Lachesis
The terror of insanity of	Mancinella
The irritability and intolerance of pain	Chamomilla
The suspicion and restlessness of	Arsenic album
The terrors of anticipation of	Argentum nitricum
The fear of death of	Aconite and Ars. alb
The sensation of tallness and superiority of	Platina
The sensation of unreality of	Medorrhinum
The sensation of two wills of	Anacardium
The indifference to loved ones of	Sepia and Phosphorus

Hahnemann said about his doctrine that

"Refute these truths, if you can, by showing a still more efficacious, certain and agreeable method than mine; refute them not by words, which we have already too much; but, if experience should prove to you, as it has done to me, that my method is the best, make use of it to save your fellow creatures and give glory to God".

He was an inveterate and flawless experimentalist. He said

"This doctrine appeals solely to the verdict of experience. Repeat experiment, it cries aloud; repeat them carefully and accurately, and you will find the doctrine confirmed at every step; and it does what no medical doctrine ever did or could do, it insists upon being judged by the results".

He based his inferences and conclusions on "inductive logic", i.e., drawing general inferences only from repeated experimentation; *'prove all things and hold fast to which is good'* was his method and motto.

HOW DOES IT WORK?

Homoeopathy works according to two basic principles. First, the principle of *'let like be cured by like'* and second, the principle of *'minimum dose'*.

Homoeopathy is based on the belief that the human body can take care of many diseases itself (except mechanical illness, which requires surgery) and that the symptoms and signs are the results of body's effort to throw off the disease. If these signs and symptoms are suppressed, the body becomes unable to use its self curing systems.

When a homoeopathic remedy is made, it is diluted with a solid (usually lactose) or a liquid (usually alcohol). It is repeatedly diluted at the scales of 1 part of remedy into 10 or 100 parts of diluent. When the diluent is a solid as lactose, the process is called '*trituration*'. In case of a liquid as alcohol being used as a diluent the two are shaken vigorously. This is called '*succussion*', and the solutions thus produced are called 'potencies'.

The strength of the remedy is expressed as 1C, 2C, 3C -------------------- 30C, 200C, when each successive dilution is made at the scale of hundred and is called *centesimal*. When the dilution scale is tenfold the system is called *decimal* and expressed as 1X, 3X --- 30X in UK, and 1D, 2D, 3D------ 30D in Europe.

As the remedy is triturated or succussed (shaken) repeatedly there comes a stage when there are very few molecules of the original remedy left in the solution. For example, when 12C dilution is made there may only be one or no molecule of the remedy left in the solution yet it would still be homoeopathically effective. The process through which a homoeopathic remedy becomes more powerful or energetic when it is serially diluted and succussed is called '*potentisation*'.

MECHANISM OF ACTION OF HOMOEOPATHIC REMEDIES

We know that homoeopathic remedies work very well as it has been proved during the last two centuries experience but we must keep two things in mind before we try to understand this. First thing, that homoeopathic remedies are not active in the molecular chemical sense that the ordinary drugs are. The Arndt-Schulz Law expresses the same principle. '*Large doses of a poisonous substance may prove lethal, smaller doses inhibit but trace doses of the same poison can actually stimulate vital cellular function*'. This has been proved in the laboratory.

To understand this principle, we need to seek help from latest development in nuclear physics. ***Avogadro's law*** states that the number of molecules in one-gram mole of a substance is 6.023×10^{-23}. This means if we dilute some remedy to 10^{-24} (12 C potency), no molecule of the original substance be present. Recent studies have shown that, the water or alcohol in which they were originally diluted might carry information (in the form of energy) about the original substance. The original substance has ***"imprinted"*** itself on to the water molecule.

The latest concept in science is that energy rather than mass is at the base of everything. The knowledge of crystal structure and function also indicates how a homoeopathic remedy associates with lactose to form new energy-rich lattices under the effect of physical grinding. By grinding or succussing an increasingly potent remedy with new diluent, more energy is built up in the molecules.

The homoeopathic remedy is given to the patient in low concentration but high ***Intrinsic Energy State***. It is this energy which is then released to stimulate various bio-energetic systems in the body. It has also been suggested by nuclear physicists that such imprinted energy patterns have self-replicating qualities. They may actually 'reproduce' in the bio-energetic systems of the body unlike other drugs are simply metabolized and excreted.

WHAT IS SO SPECIAL ABOUT HOMOEOPATHY?

1. Homoeopathy treats the patient with disease and not only the disease. It does not treat the patient in parts, rather it takes the human body as one, single, interconnected, dynamic unit, consisting of body, mind and spirit. Therefore, it is a *'whole person medicine'*. It aims at correcting the body's doctor, the 'vital force' which in turn

brings back the harmony, homeostasis or equilibrium to the normal.

2. It offers curative remedies for diseases for which others have nothing, both in chronic and acute diseases.

3. The homoeopathic remedies have been developed after repeated experiments *(provings)* on healthy, intelligent, truthful and dedicated human volunteers, and not on the animals which cannot express their signs and symptoms; especially the emotions, the subjective sensations and feelings. Experiments performed on animals and inferences thus drawn cannot be applied equally to the human beings; it seems an irrational approach. Therefore, the true or rational system is the one which utilitises the results of experiments carried out on healthy human beings for the healing of other human beings.

4. That's why no homoeopathic remedy had ever been, or will ever be declared obsolete or excluded from the materia medica due to toxic side effects; reason being the rational (natural) approach adopted in preparation.

5. The homoeopathic materia medica is very flexible, comprehensive and stable; it offers more than two thousand remedies. It has following characteristics: -

    a. The materia media offers remedies not only for preventing and curing the diseases of human beings but also for animals and birds.

    b. The remedies are almost always taken by mouth.

    c. They never produce toxic side effects in the expert hands.

    d. They can be stored for long periods without losing their activity.

    e.   For the chronic and incurable cases on long term medication, it offers better palliative remedies without any toxic side effects.

    f.   About twenty remedies can cope with most of everyday diseases and are so safe that they are ideal for self-medication and home treatment.

    g.   They can also be used as preventives.

6.   For every patient a specific remedy is selected which is capable of producing by itself a symptom-complex (artificial disease) similar to that, which it is intended to cure.

SELECTION OF REMEDY

    Selection of remedy or remedies in a case depends upon the following criteria.

    a.   Knowledge of remedies in the materia medica (the drug picture).

    b.   Knowledge of the sick patient (the disease picture).

    c.   The art and skill in matching the disease picture with the drug picture.

    d.   The causation of disease or symptom-complex.

    e.   The temperament and constitution of patient.

    f.   The pathology or disease of the patient and laboratory and other investigations.

SELECTION OF POTENCY

    Potency of the remedy is chosen on the following considerations.

    a.   The depth of action of remedy.

b. The acuteness or chronicity of case.
c. The susceptibility of the patient.
d. The plane of action expected of the remedy i.e, the physical or mental.
e. Other medicines being used by the patient concurrently.
f. Habits of patient, like alcohol abuse, smoking, tobacco chewing, drug addiction.
g. Level of intelligence of the patient.
h. Age and sex of the patient.
j. Presence of pathological changes or otherwise in the body tissues.
k. The patient is incurable or curable. According to homeopathic principle no disease is incurable; it is the patient who is curable or incurable.

HOW TO USE THIS BOOK

1. This book has been arranged in an alphabetical order to enable the reader to select the most appropriate remedy or formula, in minimum possible time and with least effort. This arrangement has made it especially valuable.

2. Most of the formulas contain three remedies, which are easy to be prepared and dispensed.

3. The first or uppermost remedy in the formula is the specific or near-specific for most of the patients corresponding to that rubric or symptom.

4. The remedies have been given in every formula according to their repertorial importance, in descending order. Therefore, most of the cases respond positively to the uppermost remedy; whereas remaining cases are cured by the lower two remedies, if used as single remedies.

5. Mostly the potencies recommended are 3x, 6x, 30 and 200. In some formulas 200 potency may be tried if 30 potency fails. The formulas with 30 potency may be repeated after every one to two hours, especially in acute cases; The 30 potency may be repeated three to four times daily; whereas 200 may be given once or twice daily, depending upon the response of the patient.

6. Lotions, ointments and shampoos or mother tinctures have been prescribed at required places.

7. Concomitant symptoms and diseases have been mentioned frequently with the chief complaint of the patient. These must be consulted to complete the '*totality*' of the case.

8. Complete names of remedies have been given at the end of the book with their abbreviations.

9. For some symptoms and diseases more than one formula have been advised. A suitable formula may be chosen out of these, according to the symptom-similarity and modalities (aggravation and amelioration).

10. Under some ailments a general formula has been given, which is suitable for majority of cases of that disorder.

11. Those fond of using single remedy or classical homeopathy, may also benefit from this work; They may easily find the single indicated remedy out of the good selected group of remedies under the relevant rubric.

12. The symptoms, signs, diseases, laboratory findings and names of organs have been given in this work, with their respective formulas, to facilitate the process of consultation.

13. The book has been arranged in repertorial fashion so that the practitioner can repertorise the case, if he desire so.

14. The *aggravations, causations*, and *ameliorations* have been presented in detailed manner. These will be of tremendous help for accurate and convenient prescribing.

15. Inter-current remedies, *Nosodes* and *Sarcodes*.

    a. Inter-current remedy is one which is given with the selected remedy but at longer intervals, to increase the curative response of the vital force. Examples are Sulfur, Carbo.veg., Opium, X-rays, etc. These remedies have been indicated below the relevant formulas, with an abbreviation of icr. These are given in the potency of 30 once daily and 200 on alternate days or weekly.

b. ***Nosodes*** are the medicinal substances, prepared from the disease products or the excretion of living organisms. ***Sarcodes*** are the medicines prepared from the secretions of healthy organisms. Nosodes and sarcodes are also written below the respective formulas. The recommended potencies are 200-1000, at weekly or fortnightly intervals; must be given in morning before 1200 hours, with a precaution that the formula or selected remedy is not to be given on the day when a nosode or sarcode is given. Commonly used nosodes are Psorinum, Syphilinum, Tuberculinum, Secale corn. Examples of sarcodes are Cholesterinum, Insulin, Thyroidin.

16. Selecting the proper potency is a very difficult and tricky affair. This book provides the most effective, reliable and verified potencies along with all the remedies.

17. Where required the cross references have been made.

18. Although the alphabetical order of the rubrics has made the consultation easy and quick, but a detailed index has been provided at the end of the book to make it more convenient and useful. The index must be repeatedly and thoroughly studied and memorized to get the best results from this work.

19. The diseases of one organ or system have been collected at one place under one heading. For example, all the eye symptoms and diseases have been listed below the rubric 'EYE'. Similarly, the ear, heart, kidney, liver and diseases of nose have been mentioned under their respective alphabets.

20.   The potencies recommended during pregnancy are 3x, 6x and 30. The remedy should not be repeated frequently during pregnancy.

21.   The readers must use a medical dictionary and a materia medica to get maximum benefit out of this book.

22.   Diseases of pregnancy, climacteric and puerperium have been mentioned separately in respective groups.

A

ABDOMEN

Distended
China	30
Carb. veg	30
Lycopod	30

Large, due to fat deposits (obesity)
Calc. carb	30
Phytolacca	30
Fucus. v	30

Large, after labor
Sepia	30
Colocynth	30
Calc. carb	30

Right-sided affection
Bryonia	30
Ars. alb	30
Lycopod	30

Left-sided affections
Lachesis	30
Palladium	30
Vespa. v	30

ABORTION

General remedies: Alet.f, Cauloph, Calc.fluor, Cimicifuga, Helonias, Kali.c, Secal.cor, Sepia, Vib.op

From debility
Alet.f	30
Chin.sulph	30
Helonias	30

Tendency to abort (habitual)
Alet.f	30
Cauloph	30
Secale.cor	30
(Sepia-200 as icr)	

From 2nd to 3rd month
Sepia	30
Vib.op	30
Sabina	30

Due to injury or over-exertion
Arnica	30
Helonias	30
Vib.op	30

After-effects of
Sabina	30
China	30
Carb.veg	30

ABSCESS. *The following formula is to be administered in low potency if the process of suppuration is to be promoted and the pus has to be drained; and in high potency if the suppuration has to be stopped.*

Calc. sulph	30
Hep. sulph	30
Merc. sol	30

About bones, joints
Aur. met	30-200
Phosphorus	30-200
Silicea	30-200

Chronic
Calc.flour	30
Merc.sol	30
Silicea	30

Injection abscess
Hep.sulph	30
Silicea	30
Thuja	30

ACIDITY *(excess of acid in stomach)*
Calc.carb	30
Nux.vom	30
Pulsatilla	30
Carb.veg	30

ACNE
Head remedies: Kali.brom, Calc.phos, Asterias.rub, Belladona, Berb. aquifol. Q

Simplex with or without pimples
Kali.brom	30
Aster.rub	30
Berb.aquifol	30

With gastric derangements
Antim.c	30
Nux.vom	30
Carb.veg	30

With menstrual irregularities
Cimicifuga	30
Pulsatilla	30
Graphite	30

ACNE, ROSACEA
1.	Ars.brom	6x
	Belladona	6x
2.	Sepia	6x
	Oophpor	6x

ACTINOMYCOSIS *(Fungal infection, abscess)*
Kali.iod	30
Nit.acid	30
Hippoz	30
(Hekla. L. as icr)	

ADDISON's DISEASE
1.	Adrenalin	30
	Calc.ars	30
	Iodum	30
2.	Ars.alb	30
	Nat.mur	30
	Arg.nit	30
	(Bacil.or Tub. as icr)	

ADENITIS *(lymph node inflammation)*
Acute
Cistus.c	30-200

Hep.sulph	30-200
Merc.sol	30-200

Chronic
1. Baryt. carb — 30
   Merc.i.r. or (Merc.cor) — 30
   Kali.iod — 30
2. Calc.carb — 30
   Phytolacca — 30
   Spongia — 30
   (Tub.or Bacil. as icr)

ADENITIS-LOCATION

Axillary
- Aster.rub — 30
- Baryt.carb — 30
- Conium — 30

Cervical(neck)
- Baryt. carb — 30
- Hep.sulph — 30
- Merc.i. r — 30

Inguinal (groin)
- Baryt. carb — 30
- Merc.sol — 30
- Nit. acid — 30

Adenoids (at posterior end of nares in throat)
- Agraphis.n — 30
- Baryt. carb — 30
- Hep.sulph — 30

ADYNAMIA-COLLAPSE *(extreme weakness and shock)*

- Ars.alb — 30
- Carb.veg — 30
- Cupr.met — 30
- (Camphor-200 single dose)

From acute diseases, mental strain
- Anacard — 30
- China. ars — 30
- Phos.acid — 30

From drugging
Carb.veg	30
Nux. vom	30
Helonias	30

From excesses, vital drains
Anacard	30
China	30
Phos.acid	30

From heat of Summer
Antim.c	30
Gelsemium	30
Nat.c	30

From jaundice
Ferr.pic	30
Pic.acid	30
Tarax	30

In aged
Conium	30
Phosphorus	30
Selenium	30

Worse from exertion, walking
Ars.alb	30
Pic.acid	30
Stannum	30

Worse in women, worn out due to hard mental and physical work, or luxury.
Helonias	30
Carb.veg	30
Cocculus	30

AGGRAVATIONS AND CAUSATIONS

Air, cold, dry
Aconite.n	30
Bryonia	30
Rhus.tox	30

Bending forward
Belladona	30
Kalmia	30

Nux.vom	30

Coitus
China	30
Kali. c	30
Phosphorus	30

Damp, living houses
Aran.d	30
Dulcamara	30
Nat. sulph	30

Erratic, shifting, changing symptoms
Ignatia	30
Kali.bich	30
Pulsatilla	30
(Tub. or Lac.can. as icr)	

Fats
Cyclamen	30
Pulsatilla	30
Carb.veg	30

Fish
Nat. sulph	30
Urtica. urens	30
Graphite	30

Grief
Phos. acid	30
Gelsemium	30
Ignatia	30

Light
Belladona	30
Nux.vom	30
Conium	30

Localised Symptoms
Ignatia	30
Kali.bich	30
Coff. c	30

Lying down
Ars.alb	30
Pulsatilla	30
Rhus.tox	30

Lying on left side
- Cactus — 30
- Spigelia — 30
- Phosphorus — 30

Lying on right side
- Mag.mur — 30
- Merc.sol — 30
- Rhus.tox — 30

Mental exertion
- Anacard — 30
- Cocculus — 30
- Gelsemium — 30

Milk
- Aethusa — 30
- Carb.veg — 30
- China — 30

Misdeed of others
- Colchicum — 30
- Staphysagria — 30
- Ignatia — 30

Mortification from an offence
- Colocynth — 30
- Lycopod — 30
- Staphysagria — 30

Motion
- Belladona — 30
- Bryonia — 30
- Nux.vom — 30

Narcotics
- Chamomilla — 30
- Nux.vom — 30
- Coff. c — 30

Night
- Ars.alb — 30
- Rhus.tox — 30
- Pulsatilla — 30

One half of body
- Chamomilla — 30
- Ignatia — 30
- Thuja — 30

Riding

Cocculus	30
Petroleum	30
Sanicula	30

Rising

Bryonia	30
Cocculus	30
Nux.vom	30

Room, heated

Glonoine	30
Merc.sol	30
Pulsatilla	30

Sedentary habits

Nux.vom	30
Anacard	30
Bryonia	30

Sitting

Bryonia	30
Rhus. tox	30
Lycopod	30

Smoking

Gelsemium	30
Ignatia	30
Nux.vom	30

Spring

Nat.mur	30
Ars.brom	30
Sarsaparilla	30

Standing

Berb.vulg	30
Cyclamen	30
Sulphur	30

Straining, overlifting, stretching

Rhus. tox	30-200
Arnica	30-200
Carbo.an	30-200
(Ruta as icr)	

Sun

Gelsemium	30

Bryonia	30
Pulsatilla	30

Sweets

Arg.nit	30
Lycopod	30
Zinc. met	30
(Medorr. as icr)	

Talking

Arg.met	30
Cocculus	30
Stannum	30

Tobacco chewing

Ars.alb	30
Verat.alb	30
Lycopod	30

Tobacco Smoking and passive smoking

Ignatia	30
Staphysagria	30
Cocculus	30

Touch

Belladona	30
China	30
Hep.sulph	30

Vital drains

China	30
Carb.veg	30
Phos.acid	30

Voice, using (speakers, singers, teachers)

Drosera	30
Phosphorus	30
Stannum	30

Warmth, heat

Bryonia	30
Pulsatilla	30
Mercurius	30

Warmth of bed

Sulphur	30
Mercurius	30
Pulsatilla	30

Weather, cold
    Causticum   30
    Nux.vom   30
    Rhus.tox   30

Weather, hot
    Belladonna   30
    Nat.mur   30
    Podophyllum   30
    (Syphil. as icr)

Wetting feet
    Rhus.tox   30
    Pulsatilla   30
    Silicea   30

ALCOHOLISM   *See Delirium*

ALOPECIA *(hair-falling) See Ringworm and Syphilis*

AMELIORATIONS

Air, cool, open
    China   30
    Lycopod   30
    Pulsatilla   30

Air, cool, must have windows open
    Arg.nit   30
    Pulsatilla   30
    Sulphur   30

Bending, double
    Colocynth   30
    Mag.phos   30
    Aloes   30

Cold
    Bryonia   30
    Ledum   30
    Phosphorus   30
    (Secal. cor. as icr)

Cold water
    Bryonia   30
    Causticum   30

Ledum	30
Drinks, warm	
Lycopod	30
Spongia	30
Ars.alb	30
Exercise	
Rhus.tox	30
Plumbum	30
Sepia	30
Expectoration	
Stannum	30
Antim. tart	30
Zinc.met	30
Fanned, being	
Carb.veg	30
China	30
Arg.nit	30
Fasting	
Anacard	30
Chelidonium	30
Ignatia	30
Feet in ice water	
Ledum	30
Secale. cor	30
Head, wrapped up warm	
Hep.sulph	30
Phosphorus	30
Silicea	30
(Psorinum as icr)	
Heat	
Ars.alb	30
Capsicum	30
Xerophyllum	30
Lying down	
Belladona	30
Bryonia	30
Nux.vom	30
Pulsatilla	30

Lying on left side
Nat.mur	30
Stannum	30
Ignatia	30
(Mur.ac as icr)	

Lying on painful side
Bryonia	30
Colocynthis	30
Pulsatilla	30

Lying on right side
Phosphorus	30
Sulphur	30
Nat. mur	30

Pressure
Bryonia	30
China	30
Pulsatilla	30

Rest
Bryonia	30
Colchicum	30
Nux.vom	30

Summer, during
Alumina	30
Calc.phos	30
Ferrum. met	30

Warmth, heat
Ars.alb	30
Hep.sulph	30
Mag.phos	30

Weather, dry
Calc.carb	30
Petroleum	30
Am. carb	30

ANAEMIA
General Formulas
1.	Carb. veg	30
	China	30

	Ferr. met	30
2.	Nat. mur	6x
	Calc. phos	6x
	Ferr. phos	6x

From menstrual derangements

Calc. carb	30
Ferr. met	30
Nat. mur	30

From nutritional disturbances

Calc. phos	30
Ferr. met	30
Nux. vom	30

From vital drains, exhausting diseases

1.	China	30
	Ferr. met	30
	Nat. mur	30
2.	Calc. phos	30
	Chin. Sulph	30
	Kali. carb	30

APPETITE-THINGS THAT DISAGREE

Butter

Carb.veg	30
Nat.mur	30
Pulsatilla	30

Cabbage

Bryonia	30
Carb.veg	30
Lycopod	30

Eggs

Ferrum. met	30
Colchicum	30
Sulphur	30

Food of any kind

Carb.veg	30
Nat.c	30
Amyg.pers	30

Milk

Calc.carb	30
Carb.veg	30

Aethusa	30

Pastry

Pulsatilla	30
Lycopod	30
Antim.c	30

Potatoes

Alumina	30
Sepia	30

APPETITE-PERVERTED CRAVINGS *(Pica)*

Excessive Desires

Acids, pickles, sour things

Ars.alb	30
China	30
Hep.sulph	30

Charcoal, coal, chalk, etc

Alumina	30
Calc.carb	30
Cicuta	30
(Psorinum. as icr)	

Coffee

Angustura	30
Ars. alb	30
Conium	30

Meat

Calc.phos	30
Mag. carb	30
Abies.n	30

Salt

Causticum	30
Phosphorus	30
Nat.mur	30

Sweets, candy

Lycopod	30
Kali.bich	30
Sulphur	30

Tea

Alumina	30
Hep.sulph	30

Thuja	30
Tobacco	
Asarum	30
Carb.veg	30
Staphysagria	30

ARTHRITIS   *See Rheumatism*

ASCARIS   *See Worms*

ASCITES   *See Oedema*

ASPHYXIA

Antim. tart	30
Hydrocy. acid	30
Neonatorum	
Antim. tart	30
Lauroc	30

ASTHENOPIA   *See Eyes, Amblyopia*

ASTHMA, *Bronchial, Cardiac*   *See Dyspnoea*

AVERSIONS   *See Appetite – Things that disagree*

AXILLA

Abscess, Acne	
Hep.sulph	30
Iridium	30
Carb.veg	30
Eczema	
Elaps	30
Nat.mur	30
Sulphur	30
Glands	*See Adenitis*
Herpes	
Carbo. an	30
Rhus.tox	30
Ars.alb	30
Sweat, profuse, offensive	
Calc.carb	30

Nit. acid 30
Tellur 30

B

BACKACHE

Rhus. tox	30
Bryonia	30
Calc.carb	30

Aching as if it would break and give out

Aesculus	30
Kalmia	30
Rhus.tox	30

Between scapulae

Calc.carb	30
Podophyllum	30
Rhus.tox	30

Bruised

Arnica	30
Hamamelis	30
Rhus.tox	30

Lancinating, drawing, tearing

Berb.vulg	30
Strychnine	30
Lycopod	30

Lancinating, extends down thighs, legs

Berb.vulg	30
Colocynthis	30
Aesculus	30

Paralytic

Cocculus	30
Kali. Phos	30
Nat.mur	30
(Silice as icr)	

Aggravation from motion, walking

Bryonia	30
Kali.c	30
Sulphur	30

Agg. at night

Merc.sol	30
Staphysagria	30
Lycopod	30

Agg.when rising from seat
　　Berb.vulg　　　　　　　　　　30
　　Causticum　　　　　　　　　　30
　　Aesculus　　　　　　　　　　　30

Amelioration. lying on back
　　Aesculus　　　　　　　　　　　30
　　Cobalt　　　　　　　　　　　　30
　　Rhus.tox　　　　　　　　　　　30

Amel. from motion, walking
　　Rhus.tox　　　　　　　　　　　30
　　Sulphur　　　　　　　　　　　 30
　　Pulsatilla　　　　　　　　　　 30

BACK, WEAKNESS

1.　Aesculus　　　　　　　　　　　30
　　China　　　　　　　　　　　　 30
　　Kali.c　　　　　　　　　　　　 30
2.　Helonias　　　　　　　　　　　30
　　Sepia　　　　　　　　　　　　 30
　　Cocculus　　　　　　　　　　　30

BAKER's ITCH (Lichen)

Lichen planus (small, flat, itching papules on wrists, legs, buccal mucosa)

1.　Sul.iod　　　　　　　　　　　　6x
　　Ars.alb　　　　　　　　　　　　6x
　　Kali.bich　　　　　　　　　　　6x
2.　Antim.c　　　　　　　　　　　　6x
　　Jugl.c　　　　　　　　　　　　 6x
　　Sulphur　　　　　　　　　　　　6x

Lichen simplex (skin lesions of solid papules with exaggerated skin markings).
　　Kreosotum　　　　　　　　　　6x
　　Lycopod　　　　　　　　　　　6x
　　Sulphur　　　　　　　　　　　6x

BARBER's ITCH *(sycosis or folliculitis of the beard or inflammation of the hair follicles)*
　　Sul.iod　　　　　　　　　　　　6x

	Thuja	6x
	Lycopod	6x

BASEDOWS DISEASE *See Goitre,*

BED SORES *(Decubitus)*

1.	Arnica		30
	Echinacea		30
	Fluor.ac		30
2.	Mur.ac		30
	Sulph.ac		30
	Carb.veg		30

BELL'S PALSY *(Paralysis of Face)*
Left side

Cadm.sulph	30
Senega	30
Gelsemium	30

Right side

Belladona	30
Causticum	30
Dulcamara	30

BILIARY COLIC *(also see colic)*

1.	Berb.vulg	30
	China	30
	Card.m	30
2.	Dioscorea	30
	Belladona	30
	Colocynthis	30

BILIOUSNESS

1.	Bryonia	30
	Chelidonium	30
	Merc. sol	30
2.	Baptisia	30
	Nat.sulph	30
	Nux.vom	30

BLADDER, DISEASES
In old men

Pop.tr	30
Copaiva	30

Staphysagria	30

Atony (also see paralysis)
Ars.alb	30
Plumbum	30
Dulcamara	30

Enuresis (urinary incontinence)
General remedy
Belladona	6x
Causticum	6x
Gelsemium	6x
Cantharis	6x

Diurnal (day time)
Causticum	6x
Equisatum	6x
Ferrum. phos	6x

Nocturnal (during night)
Belladona	30
Causticum	30
Equisatum	30

Weak or paretic sphincter of bladder
Belladona	30
Causticum	30
Gelsemium	30

Haemorrhage
Hamamelis	30
Millefolium	30
Thlaspi	30

Inflammation *(Cystitis)*
Acute
Causticum	30
Equisatum	30
Merc. cor	30

Chronic
1.	Benz.ac	30
	Cantharis	30
	Merc.cor	30
2.	Cann. sativa	30

	Ars.alb	30
	Causticum	30

BLADDER AND NECK
Irritability
1.		Benz. acid	30
		Cantharis	30
		Equisatum	30
2.		Eupat. purp	30
		Petroselinum	30
		Staphysagria	30

Irritability in women
	Eupat. purp	30
	Sepia	30
	Gelsemium	30

BLADDER, PAIN
Burning
1.		Aconite	30
		Ferrum. phos	30
		Tereb	30
2.		Uva.ursi	30
		Thuja	30
		Capsicum	30

Cutting, stitching
	Aconite	30
	Cantharis	30
	Lycopod	30

Neuralgic, spasmodic
	Belladona	30
	Lycopod	30
	Staphysagria	30

Radiating to spermatic cord
	Clematis	30
	Lith.carb	30
	Spongia	30

BLADDER, PARALYSIS
1.		Causticum	30
		Gelsemium	30

	Arnica	30
2.	Ars.alb	30
	Cantharis	30
	Equisatum	30

Weakness, inability to retain urine; dribbling

1.	Causticum	30
	Gelsemium	30
	Staphysagria	30
2.	Cann.ind	30
	Equisatum	30
	Verbascum	30

BLEPHARITIS *(inflammation of margin of eyelids)*
See Eyes

BLINDNESS *(Amaurosis)*   *See Vision*

BLOOD DISORGANISATION

Ars.alb	30
Baptisia	30
Rhus.tox	30

BLOOD

Defficiency   *See Anaemia*

Disorders remedy

Scrofularia	3x
Conium	3x
Galium.ap	3x
Hep.sulph	3x

Purifier formula

Echinacea	3x
Gunpowder	3x
Sulphur	3x

And lymphatic disorders

Kali.mur	6x
Kali.sulph	6x
Calc.sulph	6x
Nat.mur	6x

BLISTERS
Small
Ars.alb	6x
Rhus. tox	6x
Nat.mur	6x

Large
Cantharis	6x
Apis	6x
Urtica. urens	6x

BODY, as a whole
Bruised sore feeling all over
Baptisia	30
Gelsemium	30
Rhus.tox	30

Burning in various parts
Ars.alb	30
Cantharis	30
Phosphorus	30

Coldness
Aethusa	30
Baryt.mur	30
Verat.alb	30

Numbness
Aconite	30
Phosphorus	30
Secale. cor	30

Swelling (see dropsy also)
Apis	6x
Doryphora	6x
Fragaria	6x

Trembling
Agaricus.m	6x
Conium	6x
Gelsemium	6x

BONE AFFECTIONS
Condyles, epiphyses, swollen
Conchiolin	30
Rhus.tox	30

Development, slow
    Calc.phos   6x
    Calc.carb   6x
    Calc.fluor   6x

Enlargement (Acromegaly)
    Pituitrin   30
    Thyroidin   30

Exostosis
    Calc. fluor   6x
    Hekla.l   6x
    Silicea   6x

Fracture, slow union
    Calc.phos   6x
    Symphytum   6x
    Silicea   6x

Inflammation (osteitis)
    Aur.met   30
    Kali.iod   30
    Merc.sol   30

Necrosis
    Stront.c   30
    Asafoetida   30
    Phosphorus   30

Necrosis, vertebrae
    Calc.carb   30
    Nat.mur   30
    Silicea   30

Pains
    Aur.met   30
    Mezereum   30
    Mercurius   30

BOWEL OBSTRUCTION, INTUSSUSCEPTION

1. Belladona   30
    Merc.cor   30
    Nux.vom   30
2. Plumbum   30
    Opium   30

Colocynth	30

Obstruction, post-operative

Arnica	30
Belladona	30
Merc.cor	30

BRACHIALGIA *See Neuralgia*

BRADYCARDIA *(slow pulse) See Pulse*

BRAIN AFFECTIONS

ABSCEESS

Arnica	30
Iodum	30
Crot.h	30

ATROPHY (difficult thinking, concentration, weak memory)

Baryt. carb	6x
Phosphorus	6x
Iodum	6x

CONCUSSION

Arnica	30
Hypericum	30
Nat.sulph	30

INFLAMMATION (Meningitis, cerebral, acute and chronic)

Apis	30-200
Cicuta	30-200
Helleb	30-200
(Tub. as icr)	

INFLAMMATION, Cerebrospinal

1.	Belladona	30-200
	Cicuta	30-200
	Gelsemium	30-200
2.	Agaricus.m	30
	Helleb	30
	Zinc.cy	30

ISCHAEMIA (giddiness, noises in head, weak memory)

Ars.alb	6x

China		6x
Nux.vom		6x

SCLEROSIS (degeneration)

Aur.met	30
Plumb.met	30
Zinc.met	30

TUMORS

1.	Baryt. carb	30
	Conium	30
	Plumbum	30
2.	Kali.iod	30
	Hydrastis	30
	Sepia	30

BRAIN-FAG

Phos. acid	6x
Anacard	6x
Arg.nit	6x

BREATH

Cold

Carb. veg	30
Heloderma	30
Verat.alb	30

Offensive (fetor oris)

Nux.vom	30
Merc.sol	30
Pulsatilla	30

BRIGHT's DISEASE   *See Nephritis*

BROMIDROSIS *(offensive sweat)*   *See Sweat*

BRONCHIECTASIS *(bronchorrhoea, dilatation of bronchi due to bronchial obstruction and infection, with cough, muco-purulent sputum. haemoptysis and recurring pneumonia)*

Pulsatilla	30
Stannum	30

Kali.bich	30

BRONCHITIS
Acute
Bryonia	30
Ipecac	30
Hep.sulph	30

Chronic (Winter catarrh)
Am. carb	30
Carb.veg	30
Stannum	30

BRUISES   See Injuries

BUBO
Merc.i. r	30
Kali.iod	30
Nit.acid	30

BULBAR PARALYSIS *(see paralysis also)*
Guaiacum	30
Mang.ox	30
Plumbum	30

BUNIONS, *on big toe*
Benz.acid	30
Rhodendron	30
Silicea	30

BURNS, SCALDS
Cantharis	30
Causticum	30
Ars.alb	30

External applications: Calendula Q, Canth.Q, and Urtica.u. Q as lotions or ointments. Burns fail to heal or ill-effects of burns, Causticum-200

BURSITIS *(synovitis, inflammation of knee joint, House maid's knee)*
1.	Rhus.tox	30
	Bryonia	30

2. Hep.sulph   30
    Benz.acid   30
    Merc.sol   30
    Silicea   30

C

CALCULI
BILIARY (Cholilithiasis)
Berb.vulg	30
Calc.carb	30
Card.m	30
Dioscorea	30

RENAL, gravel (nephrolithiasis) See Kidney Stones

CANCER
1.	Ars.alb	30-200
	Iodum	30-200
	Thuja	30-200
	Kali.mur	30-200
2.	Condurango	30
	Asterias. rubins	30
	Kreosoteum	30
	Hydrastis	30
3.	Kali. cyan	30
	Hoang.n	30
	Pulsatilla	30

BONE
Aur.iod	30-200
Phosphorus	30-200
Symphytum	30-200

BREASTS
Carbo.an	30-200
Hydrastis	30-200
Conium	30-200

COLON
Kali.permang	30
Kali.mur	30
Urtica. urens	30

LIVER
Card.m	30
Kali.mur	30
Hydrastis	30

PAIN, to relieve
Ars.alb	30-200
Euphorbium	30-200
Hydrastis	30-200

STOMACH
Ars.alb	30-200
Condurango	30-200
Hydrastis	30-200

UTERUS
Aur.m.n	30-200
Secale. cor	30-200
Iodum	30-200

(Carcinocin, Medorrhin. Scrirrhin. as icr)

CARBUNCLE, *Anthrax, Malignant pustule*
Ars.alb	30-200
Lachesis	30-200
Silicea	30-200

CARDIAC DROPSY   *See Oedema*

CARDIAC NEUROSES
Coff. c	30
Gelsemium	30
Spigelia	30

CARDIALGIA *(pain in cardiac orifice of stomach), reflux Oesephagitis*
Arg.nit	30
Bismuth	30
Nux.vom	30
Cupr.met	30

CARDIAC ORIFICE, *contraction, reflux Oesophagitis*
Phosphorus	30
Bryonia	30
Baryt.mur	30

CARTILAGES, perichondritis *(inflammation, pain)*

Ruta	30
Arg.met	30
Belladona	30

CARIES, BONES *See Bones, Necrosis*

CATALEPSY, *Trance*

Aconite	30
Cann.ind	30
Opium	30

CATARACT

1.	Calc.fluor	30
	Euphrasia	30
	Conium	30
2.	Phosphorus	30
	Sulphur	30
	Causticum	30

CATHETERISM *(fever due to catheter)*

Aconite	30
Camphor	30
Petrosel	30

CELLULITIS

Ars.alb	30-200
Merc.i. r	30-200
Rhus.tox	30-200

CEREBRO-SPINAL MENINGITIS
See Meningitis

CHANCRE, *primary lesions*

Cinnabaris	30
Kali.iod	30
Merc.sol	30

Bleeding or phagedenic

Ars.alb	30
Mers.sol	30
Nit.acid	30

CHECKED DISCHARGES, *ill-effects, from*

Baryt. carb	30
Lobel.infl	30

		Graphite	30

Foot sweats, ill effects

1.	Baryt. carb		30
	Silicea		30
	Zinc. met		30

(Psorinum as icr)

2.	Aconite		30
	Dulcamara		30
	Rhus.tox		30

Eruptions, suppressed, ill effects

Bryonia	30
Sulphur	30
Zinc.met	30

CHEEKS, *yelloes saddle*

Sepia	30
Helonias	30
Cimicifuga	30

CHICKENPOX

Animt. tart	30
Merc.sol	30
Rhus.tox	30

CHILBLAINS *(Redness, swelling, burning and later vesicles and ulcer of skin due to cold)*

Agaricus. m	30
Pulsatilla	30
Rhus.tox	30

CHILLINESS, *Coldness*

1.	Ars.alb	30
	Calc.carb	30
	Carb.veg	30
2.	Pulsatilla	30
	Nux.vom	30
	Hep.sulph	30
3.	Silicea	30
	Merc.sol	30

CHLOASMA-*liver spots, moth patches on cheeks*
Sepia	30
Caulophylum	30
Lycopodium	30

CHLOROSIS   *See Anaemia*

CHOLERA
1.	Carb.veg	30
	Cupr.met	30
	Verat.alb	30
2.	Ars.alb	30
	Merc.cor	30
	Ipecac	30

CHOLERA INFANTUM-*Summer Complaint*
1.	Aethusa	30
	Calc.carb	30
	Podophyllum	30
2.	Ars.alb	30
	Bismuth	30
	Calc.phos	30

CHOREA, St Vitus Dance-*(widespread, arrhythmic, involuntary movements of a forcible, rapid, jerky type and have brief duration)*
Agaricus. m	30
Cupr.met	30
Calc.carb	30
Rhus.tox	30

With fright
Ignatia	30
Calc.carb	30
Nat.mur	30

With nervous disturbances
Asafoetida	30
Cocculus	30
Ignatia	30

With rhythmical motions
Tarentula Hispania	30
Causticum	30
Spigelia	30

Worse during sleep
Zizia	30
Tarentula Hispania	30

Worse face
Causticum	30
Mygale	30
Cicuta	30

CIRRHOSIS, OF LIVER   *See Liver*

CLAIRVOYANCE *(seeing things not present)*
Anacard	30
Aconite	30
Phosphorus	30

CLERGYMAN'S SORE THROAT *(Chronic, follicular inflammation of pharynx)*
Arg.nit	30
Hep.sulph	30
Phytolacca	30

CLIMACTERIC DISORDERS

BREASTS, enlarged, painful: inframammary pains
Sanguinaria	30
Bryonia	30
Cimicifuga	30

BURNING, in vertex (top of head), palms and soles
Sulphur	30
Nux.vom	30
Sanguinaria	30

FAINTING SPELLS
Glonoine	30
Lachesis	30
Sulphur	30

FALLING, of hair

Sepia	30
Arnica	30
Nat.mur	30

FATIGUE, weakness, chilliness

Bellis.p	30
Calc.carb	30
Arnica	30

FLOODING (excessive menstruation, metrorrhagia)

Trillium	30-200
Ustilago	30-200
Cimicifuga	30-200

FLUSHING

Glonoine	30
Sulphur	30
Ustilago	30

GLOBUS HYSTERICUS, hysterical tendencies

Lachesis	30
Valeriana	30
Amyl.nit	30

HEADACHE

Cimicifuga	30
Glonoine	30
Sanguinaria	30

MENTAL DEPRESSION

Cimicfuga	30
Lachesis	30
Ignatia	30

PAINS IN UTERUS

Cimicifuga	30
Sepia	30
Pulsatilla	30

PALPITATIONS

Amyl.nit	30
Calc.ars	30
Lachesis	30

SWEATING, excessive

Jaborandi	30
Sepia	30

		Hep.sulph	30

COCCYX
Injury
	Hypericum	30-200
	Arnica	30-200

Itching
	Bovista	30
	Graphites	30
	Sulphur	30

Ulcer
	Paeonia	30
	Hypericum	30

COLIC
1.	Pulsatilla	30
	Ars. alb	30
	Bryonia	30
	Carb.veg	30
2.	Lycopod	30
	Belladona	30
	Rhus.tox	30
3.	Cantharis	30
	Merc.sol	30
	China	30
	Colocynth	30

BABIES
Chamomilla	30
Aethusa	30
Mag.phos	30

BILIARY, GALL STONE
Breb.vulg	30
Calc.carb	30
China	30

CHRONIC TENDENCY
Lycopod	30
Staphysagria	30
Belladona	30

FLATULENT
Aloes	30

Staphysagria	30
Belladona	30

MENSTRUAL

Cocculus	30
Pulsatilla	30
Copaiva	30

RENAL

1.	Berb.vulg	30
	Lycopod	30
	Tereb	30
2.	Calc. carb	30
	Dioscorea	30
	Sarsaparilla	30

TOXIC (lead, copper)

Alumina	30
Opium	30
Nux.vom	30

HYPOGASTRIUM

Aloes	30
Dioscorea	30
Lycopod	30

ILEO-CECAL

Merc.cor	30
Gambogia	30
Bryonia	30

COLIC, AGGRAVATION

Bending forward

Bryonia	30
Ars.alb	30
Belladona	30

Fasting

Calc.phos	30
Colocynth	30
Nux.vom	30

COLIC, AMELIORATION

Bending double

Clocynthis	30

	Mag.phos	30
	Stannum	30

Flatus.voided per ano
	Carb.veg	30
	China	30
	Colocynthis	30

COLIC, *BILIARY*

1.	Berb.vulg		30
	Calc.carb		30
	Card.m		30
	Hydrastis		30
2.	Belladona		30
	Chionanthus		30
	Colocynthis		30

RENAL   See Kidney, Colic

COLLAPSE   *See Adynamia*
COLOR-BLINDNESS   *See Vision*
COMA

1.	Apis		30-200
	Helleborus		30-200
	Opium		30-200
2.	Baptisia		30-200
	Ailanthus		30-200
	Phos.acid		30-200

COMEDONES

	Baryt. carb	30
	Nit.acid	30
	Sulphur	30

COMPLAINTS, SYMPTOMS – TYPES OF

Appear, in small spots
	Ignatia	30
	Kali.bich	30
	Ox. acid	30

From chilling
	Aconite	30
	Dulcamara	30
	Nux.vom	30

From, over lifting, Straining, Stretching
  Arnica   30-200
  Rhus.tox   30-200
  Lycopod   30-200
Improve, then relapse continually
  Sulphur   30
  Carb.veg   30
  Calc.phos   30
In old people
  Alumina   30
  Barya.carb   30
  Conium   30

CONJUNCTIVITIS   *See Eyes*
CONDYLOMATA   *See Warts*
CONSTIPATION

  1. Alumina   30
    Opium   30
    Plumb.met   30
    Hydrastis   30
  2. Bryonia   30
    Hydrastis   30
    Naphthaline   30
    Nux.vom   30
From inertia and dryness of intestines
  Aesculus   30
  Collinsonia   30
  Plumb.met   30
In women
  Asafoetida   30
  Graphite   30
  Platinum   30
Stool, dry
  Am.mur   30
  Mag.mur   30
  Nat.mur   30
Dry, ball or dung-like
  1. Alumina   30

	Nux.vom	30
2.	Plumb.met	30
	Graphite	30

Dry, must be mechanically removed
Opium	30
Plumb.met	30
Selenium	30
Silicea	30

Frequent, uneffectual urging
Nux.vom	30
Platinum	30
Nat.mur	30

No desire or urging
Alumina	30
Bryonia	30
Opium	30

Soft stool even passed with difficulty
Platinum	30
Anacard	30
Chelidonium	30

CONSTIPATION

With piles
Aloes	30
Calc.fluor	30
Nux.vom	30

With anal prolapse
Aesculus	30
Ignatia	30
Podophylum	30

Rectal pain, persistent
Aesculus	30-200
Ignatia	30-200
Nit.acid	30-200

CONVULSIONS (also see epilepsy)

Clonic
Cupr.met	30
Nicotinum	30
Gelsemium	30

Isolated group of muscles
Cicuta	30
Stramonium	30
Strychnine	30

Worms
Cina	30
Hyoscyamus	30
Santonin	30

Puerperal Convulsions
Belladona	30-200
Cicuta	30-200
Cupr.ars	30-200

Teething, dentition, in children
Aethusa	30
Cupr. met	30
Stramonium	30

Uremic
Carbol.ac	30-200
Hydrocy. ac	30-200
Opium	30-200

CORNEA

Abscess
Hep.sulph	30
Merc.cor	30
Sulphur	30

Inflammation (Keratitis)
Aur.mur	30
Kali.bich	30
Merc.cor	30

Opacities
Cann.sat	30
Euphrasia	30
Naphthaline	30

Ulcers
Hep.sulph	30
Kali.bich	30
Calc.carb	30

Wounds
Staphysagria	30
Arnica	30
Symphytum	30

CALLOSITIES, CORNS

	Antim.crud	30
	Nit.acid	30
	Thuja	30

CORYZA

Dry, stuffy colds

	Hep.sulph	30
	Kali.bich	30
	Nux.vom	30

Fluent, watery

	Ars.alb	30
	Sabadilla	30
	Nux.vom	30

Periodic

	Ars.alb	30
	China	30
	Nat.mur	30

With thick mucus

	Hep.sulph	30
	Kali.bich	30
	Merc.sol	30

Cough

	Belladona	30
	Cepa	30
	Sticta	30

Headache

	Bryonia	30
	Gelsemium	30
	Nux.vom	30

Hoarseness, aphonia

	Causticum	30
	Hep.sulph	30
	Phosphorus	30

Infants, with snuffles

	Chamomilla	30
	Hep.sulph	30

Phosphorus		30

Infants, with snuffles

Chamomilla	30
Nux.vom	30
Sambucus	30

Inflammation, chronic, atrophic (sicca)

Alumina	30
Hep.sulph	30
Lycopod	30

Inflammation, chronic, catarrhal

Alumina	30
Hydrastis	30
Merc.sol	30

COUGH

Dry

Aconite	30
Causticum	30
Bryonia	30
Spongia	30

Chronic

Allium. sat	30
Spongia	30
Drosera	30

Hoarse, hollow, metallic

Arum.tri	30
Hep.sulph	30
Causticum	30
Phosphorus	30

COWPERITIS

1.	Cann.sat	30
	Hep.sulph	30
	Sabal.s	30
2.	Merc.cor	30
	Petrosel	30
	Silicea	30

CRACKED LIPS, ULCERATIONS

Kali.mur	30

Ars.alb	30
Graphite	30

CRAMPS

Cupr.met	30
Mag.phos	30
Calc.phos	30

CRETINISM

Anacard	30
Baryt.carb	30
Thyroidin	30

CYANOSIS *(blue colour of skin, lips, tongue)*

1.	Ars.alb	30
	Carb.veg	30
	Rhus.tox	30
2.	Laurocerasus	30
	Digitalis	30
	Antim.tart	30

CYSTITIS   *See Bladder*

CYSTS, OVARIAN

Aur.iod	30
Colocynth	30
Lycopod	30

CYSTS, Sebaceous

Baryt. carb	30
Conium	30
Kali.iod	30

CYSTIC TUMORS

Baryt.carb	30
Iodum	30
Kali.brom	30

D

DANDRUFF   *See Seborrhoea*

DEAFNESS

General formula for all types
- Agraphis. n   30
- Chenopodium   30
- Chin. Sulph   30

Due to adenoids or enlarged tonsils
- Agraphis.n   30
- Baryt.carb   30
- Merc.sol   30

Catarrh (eustachean, middle ear)
- Hep.sulph   30
- Kali.mur   30
- Pulsatilla   30

Human voice, difficult to hear
- Chenopodium   30
- Calc.carb   30
- Phosphorus   30

Old age
- Kali. mur   30
- Merc. dulcis   30
- Phosphorus   30

Scrofulous diathesis
- Sulphur   30
- Aethiops   30
- Mezer   30

DEBILITY   *See Adynamia*

DECUBITUS   *See Bed Sores*

DELIRIUM *(Psychological disorders)*

Alcoholic (delirium tremens)
- Agaricus. m   30
- Nux.vom   30

Stramon		30
Destructive (barks, bites, strikes etc)		
	Belladona	30-200
	Stramon	30-200
	Verat.alb	30-200
Lascivious (becomes naked)		
	Cantharis	30-200
	Hyoscyamus	30-200
	Sramonium	30-200
Loquacity, talks incessantly		
	Belladona	30-200
	Hyoscyamus	30-200
	Stramonium	30-200

DELIVERY, EASY *(three times daily during last two months)*

	Mag.phos	6x
	Calc.phos	6x
	Klai.phos	6x
	Calc.fluor	6x

DEMENTIA *(Alzheimer's disease)*

	Anacard	30-200
	Phos.acid	30-200
	Cann.ind	30-200

DENGUE FEVER *(Acute epidemic infectious disease by a virus with weakness, joint and muscle pain, lymph node involvement and leukopenia)*

	Eupat.prf	30
	Gelsemium	30
	Rhus.tox	30

DENTITION

In children, teething difficult, delayed		
	Calc.phos	6x
	Chamomilla	6x
	Kreosotum	6x
In adults (wisdom tooth)		
	Silicea	30
	Hydrastis	30
	Symphytum	30

(Aur.met. as icr)

DEPRESSION

	Ignatia	30-200
	Staphysagria	30-200
	Gelsemium	30-200

Obstinate cases

	Kali.bich	30
	Arg.nit	30
	Kali.ars	30

DERMATITIS *See Skin*

DIABETES INSIPIDUS

	Lycopod	30
	Nat.mur	30
	Uran.nit	30

DIABETES MELLITUS

1.		Ars.brom	30
		Syz.jamb	30
		Uran.nit	30
2.		Phos.acid	30
		Lycopod	30
		Nat.sulph	30
		(Seacal.cor 200 as icr)	

DIAPHRAGM *(inflammation, irritation)*

	Bryonia	30
	Cactus	30
	Nux.vom	30

DIARRHOEA-DYSENTERY

General formula

	Chin.ars	30
	Merc.cor	30
	Colocynth	30
	Verat.alb	30

From emotional excitement, fright

	Aconite	30

Gelsemium	30
Phos.acid	30

From fats

Pulsatilla	30
Cyclamen	30
Kali.mur	30

From fruits

Ars.alb	30
Bryonia	30
Podophyllum	30

From gastric derangements

Antim.crud	30
Nux.vom	30
Pulsatilla	30

From hot weather

China	30
Bryonia	30
Podophyllum	30

From intestinal atony, debelity

Arg. nit	30
China	30
Ferr. phos	30

From milk

Aethusa	30
Mag. carb	30
Nat. carb	30

From typhoid fever

Ars.alb	30
Baptisia	30
Rhus.tox	30

From vegetables, melons

Ars.alb	30
Calc.phos	30
Merc.cor	30
(Sulphur as icr)	

Infants(dentition)   *See Dentition*

In old people

Carb.veg	30

China	30
Sulphur	30
(Opium. as icr)	

DIARRHOEA, TYPE OF STOOL

Bloody

Cantharis	30
Ipecac	30
Merc.cor	30

Blood streaked

Aloes	30
Merc.cor	30
Sulphur	30

Debilitating (weakening)

Ars.alb	30
China	30
Verat.alb	30

Fermented, flatulent

Arg.nit	30
Sulphur	30
Verat.alb	30

Gelatinous, jelly like

Aloes	30
Colocynth	30
Rhus.tox	30

Involuntary

Aloes	30
Gelsemium	30
Phos.acid	30

Rice-water

Ars.alb	30
Jatropha	30
Verat.alb	30

Sudden, cannot wait

Aloes	30
Crot.tig	30
Sulphur	30

DIPHTHERIA

1.	Ars.alb	30
	Merc.cyn	30
	Kali.bich	30
2.	Belladona	30
	Lachesis	30
	Phytolacca	30

DIPLOPIA *(double vision)* — *See Eyes*

DROPSY — *See Oedema*

DROWSINESS, *after meals*

China	30
Lycopod	30
Staphysagria	30

DRUGS, DIETS-ABUSE

In general

Nux.vom	30
Aloes	30
Hydrastis	30

Digitalis

China	30
Nit.acid	30
Cratagus	30

Iron

Hep.sulph	30
Pulsatilla	30
China	30

Narcotics

Avena.sat	30
Cann.ind	30
Chamomilla	30

Quinine

Ars.alb	30
Pulsatilla	30
Carb.veg	30

Salt

Phosphorus	30

Ars.alb	30
Carb.veg	30

Sugar

Merc.v	30
Nat.phos	30

Tea

Ars.alb	30
Gelsemium	30
Nux.vom	30

DUODENUM

Inflammation (Duodenitis)

Ars.alb	30
Lycopod	30
Kali.bich	30
(Nux. vom as icr)	

Ulceration

Kali.bich	30
Symphytum	30
Uran.nit	30

DYSENTERY *See Diarrhoea*

Merc.cor	30
Podophyllum	30
Ars.alb	30
(Sulphur as icr)	

DYSMENORRHOEA *(painful menstruation)*

Pulsatilla	30
Cimicifuga	30
Mag.phos	30

Irregular

Belladona	30
Pulsatilla	30
Senecio	30

Premature

Mag.phos	30
Calc.carb	30
Xanthox	30

Spasmodic, with uterine congestion

Belladona	30

Sabina	30
Cimicifuga	30

DYSPEPSIA *(indigestion)*

Bryonia	30
Carb.veg	30
Nux.vom	30

Abuse of drugs, tea, tobacco, condiments

Nux.vom	30
Carb.veg	30
Sulphur	30

Aged, debilitated

Bryonia	30
Carb.veg	30
Lycopod	30

Beer

Kali.bich	30
Bryonia	30
Nux.vom	30

Dietetic indiscretions

Bryonia	6x
Carb.veg	6x
Nux.vom	6x
Pulsatilla	6x

Excesses

China	30
Nux.vom	30
Carb.veg	30

Fatty food

Carb.veg	30
Cyclamen	30
Pulsatilla	30

Flatulent food

China	30
Lycopod	30
Pulsatilla	30

Milk

Aethusa	30
Calc.carb	30

Sulphur	30

Sedentary life

Nux.vom	30
Carb.veg	30
Lycopod	30

Tea

China	30
Dioscorea	30
Thuja	30

Tobacco

Nux.vom	30
Abies. nigra	30
Sepia	30

DYSPEPSIA-SYMPTOMS

Acidity

Calc.carb	30
Robinia	30
Nux.vom	30

Digestion, weak, slow

Ars.alb	6x
Bryonia	6x
Carb.veg	6x
Pulsatilla	6x

Distress from simplest food

Carb.veg	6x
Hep.sulph	6x
Nux.vom	6x

Eructations, foul

Arnica	6x
Carb.veg	6x
Pulsatilla	6x

Flatulent distention of stomach

1.	Carb.veg	6x
	Lycopod	6x
	Pulsatilla	6x
2.	Nux.vom	6x
	Asafoetida	6x
	Colchicum	6x

Heartburn, pyrosis
    Arg.nit   6x
    Bryonia   6x
    Calc.carb   6x

Nausea, Vomiting
    Ars.alb   6x
    Bryonia   6x
    Pulsatilla   6x
    Nux.vom   6x

Pain, immediately after eating
    Carb.veg   6x
    Kali.bich   6x
    Lycopod   6x

Pain, several hours after eating
    Agaricus. m   6x
    Nux.vom   6x
    Pulsatilla   6x

Palpitation of the heart
    Cactus   6x
    Carb. veg   6x
    Nux. vom   6x

Regurgitation of food
    Alumina   6x
    Carb. veg   6x
    Ipecacc   6x

Vertigo
    Pulsatilla   6x
    Gratiola   6x
    Nux.vom   6x
    Carb.veg   6x

DYSPHAGIA *(Difficulty in swallowing)*
    Asafoetida   6x
    Ignatia   6x
    Nux. moschata   6x

DYSPNOEA, *difficult breathing, Asthma, bronchial*
Aggravation by lying down
    Ars.alb   6x

Digitalis	6x
Pulsatilla	6x

Agg. by sitting up

Carb.veg	6x
Spongia	6x
Digitialis	6x

Agg. by walking

Aconite	6x
Ipecac	6x
Nat.mur	6x

Agg. from working

Calc.carb	30
Nat.mur	30
Sepia	30

Relief from expectoration

Antim.tart	30
Kali.bich	30
Zinc.met	30

Relief from sitting up

Ars.alb	30
Sambucus	30
Nat. sulph	30

Gasping

Ipecac	30
Phosphorus	30
Sambucus	30

Rattling

Antim.tart	30
Bromium	30
Ipecac	30

Suffocative

Antim.tart	30
Grindelia	30
Ipecac	30

DYSPONEA-*Cardiac, cardiac asthma*

1.	Aconite. fer	30
	Cactus	30

	Glonoine	30
2.	Aur.met	30
	Iodum	30
	Lachesis	30

DYSURIA *(Painful, difficult urination)*

Cantharis	6x
Staphysagria	6x
Merc.cor	6x

Pregnancy and after

Equisatum	30
Berb.vulg	30

Newly married women: (honey moon cystitis)

Staphysagria - (30)

With prostatic or uterine diseases

Conium	30
Staphysagria	30
Helonias	30

Feeble stream

Hep.sulph	30
Merc.cor	30
Clematis	30

E

EAR, AFFECTIONS *See External auditory canal, Earache, Otitis, Otalgia*

EARACHE, *pain in ear*
Pulsating, throbbing

Belladona	30
Ferrum. phos	30
Glonoine	30
Merc.sol	30

ECCHYMOSES *(extravasation of blood into subcutaneous tissue, discoloring the skin; also see black eye)*

1.
Arnica	30
Ledum	30
Sulph.acid	30

2. Calendula-Q and Ledum-Q-ointment or lotion for external application.

ECLAMPSIA, *Puerperal convulsions (a disease occurring in pregnancy, characterized by edema, sodium retention, convulsions and coma)*

Belladona	30-200
Cicuta	30-200
Cupr.ars	30-200

ECTROPION *See Eyes*

ECZEMA *See Skin*

ELEPHANTIASIS

Ars.alb	30
Hydrocotyle	30
Myristica. s	30

EMISSIONS *(nocturnal pollutions; sexual debility)*

1. Iridium-30 is the head remedy
2.
Avena sat.	6x
Cantharis	6x

Staphysagria	6x

With brain-fag, weak legs and backache

Phos.acid	30
China	30
Staphysagria	30

With emissions diurnal, straining at stool

China	6x
Nuphar. luteum	6x
Phos.acid	6x

With emissions, premature (premature ejaculation)

Agnus.castus	Q or 6x
China	6x
Graphite	6x

With erections deficient

Agnus. castus	Q or 6x
Conium	6x
Lycopod	6x

With irritability, despondency, depression

Aur.met	30
Calc.carb	30
Nux.vom	30

EMPHYSEMA *See Lungs*

EMPYEMA *See Pleurae*

ENCEPHALITIS LETHARGICA *(Sleeping sickness)*

Ars.alb	30
Atoxyl	30

ENDOCARDITIS *See Heart*

ENDOCERVICITIS *See Uterus*

ENDOMETRITIS *See Uterus*

ENTERALGIA *See Colic*

ENTERITIS *See Diarrhea*

ENTROPION *See Eyes*

ENURESIS *See Urine, Bladder*
EPIDIDYMITIS *See Testicles*
EPILEPSY

Grand Mal, Petit mal
Belladona	30
Cupr.met	30
Aethusa	30

From fright, emotional causes
Arg.nit	30
Ignatia	30
Chamomilla	30

From injury
Conium	30
Cupr.met	30
Nat.sulph	30
(Melilotus-200 as icr)	

From worms
Cina	30
Stannum	30
Teucrium	30

In children
Aethusa	30
Belladona	30
Cupr.met	30

Preceded by sudden cry
Cupr.met	30
Hydrocy.ac	30
Belladona	30

Status epilepticus
Aconite	30
Belladona	30
Oenanthe	30

EPIPHORA *(a persistent overflow of tears, due to excessive secretion or impeded flow)*
Merc.per or Merc.sol	30
Nat.mur	30

Hep.sulph	30

EPISTAXIS *See Nose*
EPITHELIOMA
Ars.alb	30
Condurango	30
Thuja	30

EROTOMANIA *See Mania*
ERUCTATIONS *See Dyspepsia*
ERYSIPELAS
1.	Arnica	30
	Cantharis	30
	Rhus.tox	30
2.	Apis	30
	Belladona	30
	Crot. tig	30

Constitutional tendency
Graphite	30
Sulphur	30
Lachesis	30
(Psorinum. as icr)	

Facial
Belladona	30
Euphorbium	30
Graphite	30

Recurrent
Graphite	30
Rhus.tox	30
Sulphur	30

ERYTHEMA
Inertrigo (Chaffing)
Merc.sol	30
Petroleum	30
Sulphur	30

Multiforme
Antipyrine	30
Boracic. acid	30

Copaiva	30

Simplex

Cantharis	30
Merc.sol	30
Rhus.tox	30

EUSTACHEAN DEAFNESS *See Deafness*
EXOPHTHALMIC GOITRE *See Goitre*
EXOSTOSES *See Bones*
EXTERNAL AUDITORY CANAL, AFFECTIONS

Boils, pimples

Merc.sol	30
Silicea	30
Belladona	30

Digging and scratching into

Cina	30
Sulphur	30
Belladona	30
(Psorinum. as icr)	

Inflammation and pain

Merc.sol	30
Pulsatilla	30
Tellurium	30

Itching

Pulsatilla	30
Sulphur	30
Tellurium	30
(Psorinum. as icr)	

Sensation, as if heat emanated from

Aethusa	30
Causticum	30
Belladona	30

Sensation, as if obstructed

Pulsatilla	30
Verbascum	30

EYES

Merc.sol 30

Agglutination

Euphrasia 30
Merc.sol 30
Graphite 30

Catarat   See Cataract

Drooping (ptosis, paralysis of eyelids)

Causticum 30
Gelsemium 30
Plumbum 30

Dryness

Aconite 30
Belladona 30
Graphite 30

Ectropion (eversion or outward turning of eyelids and eyelashes)

Apis 30
Graphite 30
Thiosinaminum 30

Entropion (inward turning of eyelids and eyelashes)

Borax 30
Nat.mur 30
Graphite 30
Tellurium 30

Epiphora   See Epiphora

EYELIDS, GROWTHS

Chalazae, trasal tumors

Conium 6x
Staphysphagria 6x
Thuja 6x

Cysts, sebaceous

Benz.acid 30
Calc.fluor 30
Staphysagria 30

Granular lids (Trachoma)

	Alumina	30
	Euphrasia	30
	Thuja	30

Pterygium   *See Pterygium*

Styes (Hordeolum)

	Pulsatilla	30
	Staphysagria	30
	Thuja	30

Inflammation of eye lid margin (Blepharitis)

Acute

	Euphrasia	30
	Merc.sol	30
	Pulsatilla	30

Chronic

	Arg.nit	30
	Borax	30
	Staphysagria	30

Redness

	Antim.crud	30
	Belladona	30
	Merc.cor	30

F

FACE APPEARANCE
Anaemic
Ars.alb	30
Calc.phos	30
Ferrum. phos	30

Bloated, puffy
Ars.alb	30
Merc.cor	30
Phos	30

Blue, livid(cyanosis)
Ars.alb	30
Carb.veg	30
Sambucus	30

Blue rings, around eyes
China	30
Phos. acid	30
Staphysagria	30

Brown spots, on
Cauloph	30
Sepia	30

Hippocratic (sickly, sunken, deathly cold)
Ars.alb	30
Carb.veg	30
Verat.alb	30

Jaundiced, yellow
Chelidonium	30
Chionanthus	30
Sepia	30

Pale
Ars.alb	30
Carb.veg	30
Merc.cor	30

FACE, BONES
Caries (exostosis, inflammation)
Aurum.met	30
Fluor.acid	30

Hekla.l 30
Pains
Aurum.met 30
Hep.sulph 30
Merc.sol 30

FACE, CHEEKS
Bites, when chewing, talking
Ignatia 6x
Causticum 6x
Oleum animale 6x
Eruptions
Antin.crud 6x
Ledum 6x
Mezereum 6x

FACE, CHIN, *eruptions*
Graphite 6x
Hep.sulph 6x
Antim.crud 6x

FACE *Acne*   *See Acne*
Comedones   *See Comedones*
Erysipelas 30
Apis 30
Cantharis 30
Rhus.tox 30
Herpes
Dulcamara 30
Nat.mur 30
Rhus.tox 30
Lentigo (Frackles)
Mur.acid 30
Lycopod 30
Sulphur 30
Pustules
Calc.sulph 30
Merc.sol 30
Hep.sulph 30
Spots, copper colored
Carbo.an 6x

Lycopod	6x
Benz.acid or Nit.acid	6x

Whiskers, eruptions, falling out, itching

Hep.sulph	6x
Selenium	6x
Calc.carb	6x

PROSOPALGIA   *See Neuralgia*
FACE, SENSATIONS

Burning, heat

Ars.alb	6x
Capsicum	6x
Sulphur	6x

Formication, numb, tingling, crawling

Aconite	6x
Platina	6x
Nux.vom	6x

FAINTING   *See Syncope*
FEARS

Being carried or raised

Borax	30
Bryonia	30
Sanicula	30

Crossing streets, crowds, excitement

Aconite	30
Hydrocy.ac	30
Platina	30

Death, fatal diseases, impending evils

Aconite	30-200
Aur. met	30-200
Platina	30-200

People (Anthropophobia)

Aur.met	30
Baryt.carb	30
Sepia	30

Stage fright

Gelsemium	30
Anacard	30
Arg.nit	30

Water (Hydrophobia)
Belladona	30-200
Hyoscyamus	30-200
Stramonium	30-200

FELON *(Whitlow, Panaritium)*
Bryonia	30
Dioscorea	30
Hep.sulph	30

FEVER

1. *Cold sponging with normal tap water is very effective.*
2. *Pyrogenium 200 is required in most of the cases.*
3. *Start the treatment with formula a or b or both if required. Majority of the cases are cured by these. In rest of the cases repertorise the case with the help of following group remedies.*
4. *Search for the nosode required, if any.*

a.	Belladona	30
	Rhus.tox	30
	Gelsemium	30
	Baptisia	30
b.	Ferr, phos	30
	Kali.mur	30
	Nat.mur	30

FEVER, *with colicky pain in abdomen and foul-smelling stool*
China	30
Merc.sol	30
Baptisia	30

With eruptions like Measles, Chicken-Pox
Ailanthus	30
Belladona	30

Euphrasia	30

With tonsillitis

Belladona	30
Phytolacca	30
Kali.iod	30

With influenza

Ars.alb	30
Gelsemium	30
Eupat.perf	30

Malaria, with shaking chill

Nat.mur	30
Ipecac	30
Chin.sulph	30

Septic

Ars.alb	30
Echinacea	30
Rhus.tox	30
(Pyrogenium as icr)	

Due to vaccination

Merc.sol	30
Hep.sulph	30
Thuja	30

FIBROID, *tumors*   See Tumors

FISTULA, *dentalis*   See Teeth

FLATULENCE   See Dyspepsia, Indigestion

FRACTURES   See Bones

FRACKLES *(lentigo)*   See Face

FUNGAL INFECTIONS   See Actinomycosis, Pityriasis, Ringworm

FURUNCLE *(boil)*

Belladona	30
Hep.sulph	30
Arnica	30
(Mercurius as icr)	

Recurrent
Arnica	30
Calc.pic	30
Hep.sulph	30

G

GAIT DISORDERS

Ataxic   *(See Locomotor Ataxia)*

Arg.nit	30
Secal.cor	30
Nux.vom	30

Sluggish, Slow

Gelsemium	30
Phosphorus	30
Causticum	30

Staggering, unsteady

Baryt.mur	30
Gelsemium	30
Zinc.met	30

Walking, child slow to learn

Baryt.carb	6x
Calc.phos	6x
Nat.mur	6x

Drags feet, when walking

Mygale	6x
Nux.vom	6x
Tabacum	6x

Stumbles easily, when walking

Agaricus. m	6x
Phos.acid	6x
Belladona	6x

GALACTORRHOEA *(milk, too profuse)*
                         See Lactation

GALL-STONES   *See Calculi, Biliary*

GALL-STONES, COLIC   *See Colic, Biliary*

GANGLION, *on back of wrist*

Benz.acid	6x
Ruta	6x
Silicea	6x

GANGRENE
1.	Secale.cor	30
	Ars.alb	30
	Carb.veg	30
2.	Echinacea	30
	Euphorbium	30
	Lachesis	30

Senile
Ars.alb	30
Cepa	30
Secal.cor	30

Traumatic
Arnica	30
Lachesis	30
Sulph. acid	30

GAS FUMES - *ill effects*
Am. carb		30
Belladona	30	
Coff. c	30	

GASTRIC PAIN
Burning, as from ulcer
Ars.alb	6x
Carb.veg	6x
Nux.vom	6x
Sulphur	6x

Crampy, colicky
Arg.nit	6x
Bismuth	6x
Carb.veg	6x
Colocynth	6x

Cutting, paroxysmal, spasmodic
Bryonia	6x
Chin.ars	6x
Colocynth	6x
Cupr.acet	6x

Epigastric (pit of stomach)
Abies.n	6x

Dioscorea	6x
Hydrastis	6x
Nux.vom	6x

Gnawing, hungry-like

Arg.nit	6x
Pulsatilla	6x
Uran.nit	6x

Aggravation
Empty stomach

Anacard	6x
Petroleum	6x
Cina	6x

From food

Arg.nit	6x
Bryonia	6x
Nux.vom	6x

Amelioration
From bending backward, standing erect

Dioscorea	30
Belladona	30

From eating

Anacard	30
Chelidonium	30
Petroleum	30

From pressure

Plumb.met	30
Fluor.acid	30
Bryonia	30

GASTRITIS
Acute

Ars.alb	6x
Nux.vom	6x
Belladona	6x
Pulsatilla	6x

Acute, from alcohol abuse

Ars.alb	30
Cupr.met	30
Nux.vom	30

Acute, with intestinal involvement
    Ars.alb 30
    Baptisia 30
    Cupr.met 30

Chronic, inflammation of stomach
    Nux.vom 30
    Physostigma 30
    Rhus.tox 30

GLEET *(Chronic Gonorrhoea)*
    Agnus.castus 30
    Cann.sat 30
    Thuja 30

Ophthalmia
    Aconite 6x
    Belladona 6x
    Merc.cor 6x

Orchitis, epididymitis
    Spongia 30
    Clematis 30
    Pulsatilla 30

Prostatic involvement
    Thuja 30
    Capsicum 30
    Pareira.b 30

Rheumatism
    Merc.cor 30
    Phytolacca 30
    Thuja 30

Stricture, Urethra
    Thuja 30
    Clematis 30
    Mercurius 30

Suppression, ill-effects
    Agnus. castus 30
    Pulsatilla 30
    Thuja 30

GLOSSITIS *(Inflammation of tongue)*   *See Tongue*

GOITRE, *Hyperthyroidism, exophthalmic*

1.	Belladona	6x
	Calc.carb	6x
	Spongia	6x
2.	Bromium	6x
	Iodum	6x
	Hydrastis	6x

Hypothyroidism (Basedow's disease)

1.	Belladona	6x
	Calc.carb	6x
	Iodum	6x
2.	Cactus	30
	Glonoine	30
	Thyroidin	30
3.	See Myxoedema also	

GONORRHOEA *(specific urethritis)*

Acute inflammation
Aconite	30
Cann.sat	30
Gelsemium	30

Adenitis, lymphangitis
Anacard	30
Cann.ind	30
Merc.sol	30

Chronic, Subacute Stage
Pulsatilla	30
Sulphur	30
Thuja	30

Chronic   See Gleet

GONORRHOEA, DISCHARGE

Bloody
Cantharis	30
Merc.cor	30
Millefolium	30

Milky, glairy, mucus
Cann.sat	30

	Hydrastis	30
	Petroleum	30

Muco-purulent, yellowish-green
	Arg.nit	30
	Causticum	30
	Hep.sulph	30

GOUT

1.		Bryonia	30
		Ledum	30
		Rhus.tox	30
2.		Nux.vom	6x
		Colchicum	6x
		Merc.sol	6x

GUMS

Bleeding, easily
	Ars.alb	30
	Carb.veg	30
	Merc. vivus	30

Bleeding, after tooth extraction
	Hamamelis	30
	Kreosotum	30
	Phosphorus	30

Inflammation(gumboil)
	Aconite	30
	Hekla.l	30
	Merc.sol	30

Painful, after tooth extraction
	Arnica	30
	Sepia	30
	Hypericum	30

Painful, sore, sensitive, gingivitis
	Carb.veg	30
	Kreosotum	30
	Merc.cor	30

Pyorrhoea alveolaris   See Pyorrhoea alveolaris

Scorbutic (soft, spongy, receding)
	Ars.alb	30

Carb.veg	30
Staphysagria	30

Ulceration
Merc.cor	30
Kreosotum	30
Phosphorus	30

H

HEADACHE – CAUSES

Catarrh
	Cepa	30
	Hydrastis	30

Catarrh suppressed
	Kali. bich	30
	Belladona	30
	(Lach. as icr)	

Constipation
	Aloes	30
	Bryonia	30
	Nux. vom	30

Emotional disturbances
1.	Gelsemium	30
	Iganatia	30
	Pic. acid	30
2.	Arg. nit	30
	Coff. c	30
	Phos. Acid	30

Eye-strain
	Nat. mur	6x
	Ruta	6x
	Gelsemium	6x

Castro-intestinal derangements
1.	China	30
	Iris. v	30
	Pulsatilla	30
2.	Nux. vom	30
	Bryonia	30
	Carb. veg	30

Mental exertion or exhaustion
1.	Arg. nit	30
	Coff. c	30
	Gelsemium	30
2.	Kali. phos	30
	Anacard	30
	Nux. vom	30

Sunlight or heat

Glonoine	30
Belladona	30
Gelsemium	30

Tobacco

Ignatia	6x
Nux. vom	6x
Gelsemium	6x

HEADACHE – LOCATION

Frontal

Belladona	30
Hydrastis	30
Nux.vom	30

Occipitial

Bryonia	30
Cocculus	30
Gelsemium	30

Temples

Belladona	30
Anacard	30
Glonoine	30

Vertex (Crown of head)

Cactus	6x
Cimicifuga	6x
Phos. Acid	6x
(Sulph. as icr)	

HEADACHE – TYPES

Anaemic

China	6x
Ferr. phos	6x
(Phos. as icr)	

Chronic

Arg. nit	6x
Cocculus	6x
Zinc. met	6x
(Psorin. as icr)	

Chronic, of school grils

Calc. phos	6x

	Kali. phos	6x
	Nat. mur	6x

Chronic, sedentary persons

	Arg. nit	6x
	Bryonia	6x
	Nux. vom	6x

Gastric, bilious

1.	Bryonia		6x
	Iris. v		6x
	Nux. vom		6x
2.	Arg. nit		6x
	Plusatilla		6x
	Sanguinaria		6x

Hysterical

	Coff. c	30
	Ignatia	30
	Platina	30

HEADACHE-CONCOMITANTS

Arterial excitement

	Belladona	30
	Glonoine	30
	Verat. v	30

Constipation

	Bryonia	30
	Hydrastis	30
	Nux. vom	30

Exhaustion, asthenia

	Ars. Alb	30
	Gelsemium	30
	China	30

Eyes, visual disturbances, before or during

	Cyclamen	30
	Gelsemium	30
	Iris. v	30

Irritability

	Broynia	30
	Chamomilla	30
	Ignatia	30

HEART DISEASES

ACTION, VIOLENT, LABORED
Belladona	30
Cactus	30
Glonoine	30

DEBILITY, WEAKNESS (heart failure)
Coff. c	30
Digitails	30
Glonoine	30

NERVOUS
Iberis	30
Naja	30
Spigelia	30

WITH DROPSY OF LEGS OR FEET
Coff. c	30
Ars.alb	30
Cactus	30
Digitails	30

DEGENERATION, FATTY
Ars.alb	30
Baryt.carb	30
Phytolacca	30

INFLAMMATION (endocarditis)
Aconite	30
Cactus	30
Spigelia	30

RHEUMATIC DISORDERS
Rhus.tox	30
Bryonia	30
Spigelia	30

Pericarditis

Acute
Ars.alb	30
Bryonia	30
Spigelia	30

Chronic
Aur.iod	30
Calc.flour	30
Kali.carb	30

Rheumatic

	Colchicum	30
	Spigelia	30
	Rhus.tox	30

Heart, Pain *(Angina pectoris)*

1.	Cactus	3x
	Golonine	3x
2.	Belladona	3x
	Coff. c	3x

From organic heart disease

Cactus	1x-3x
Cratagus	1x-3x
Ars.alb	1x-6x

From tobacco

Nux.vom	30
Spigelia	30
Staphysagria	30

Praecordial oppression, anxiety, heaviness

1.	Cactus	30
	Ars.alb	30
	Pulsatilla	30
2.	Cratagus	30
	Glonoine	30
	Passiflora	30

Shooting down left shoulder, arm to fingers

Cactus	30
Kalmia	30
Rhus.tox	30

Heart, Palpitations

Cactus	1x-3x
Glonoine	1x-3x
Passiflora	1x-3x

Anaemia, vital drains, with

China	6x
Nat.mur	6x
Phos.acid	6x

Dyspepsia, with

Carb.veg	6x

Pulsatilla	6x
Nux.vom	6x
Lycopod	6x

Tobacco

Ars.alb	6x
Gelsemium	6x
Nux.vom	6x
Strophanthus	6x

Palpitations-Concomitants

Dyspnoea

Cactus	30
Glonoine	30
Spongia	30

With flatulence

Arg.nit	30
Carb.veg	30
Nux.vom	30
Cactus	30

With pain, praecordial

Cactus	30
Coff. c	30
Spigelia	30

With sleeplessness

Coca	30
Ignatia	30
Spigelia	30

Palpitations-Aggravation

After eating

Calc.carb	6x
Lycopod	6x
Nux.vom	6x
Pulsatilla	6x

From lying on left side

Cactus	30
Phosphorus	30
(Lach.as icr)	

From lying on right side

Alumen	30

                   Arg.nit   30

HART, Valvular diseases *See Valvular diseases*

HEMETEMESIS *(vomiting of blood from stomach)*
        1.   Mag.mur   30
              Millefolium   30
              China   30
        2.   Ars.alb   30
              Carb.veg   30
              Ipecac   30

HEMATURIA   *See Urine*
HEMOGLOBINURIA   *See Urine*
HEMOPHILIA
        1.   Hamamelis   30
              Phosphorus   30
              Secal.cor   30
        2.   Crot.h   30
              Lachesis   30
              Phosphorus   30

HEMORRHAGES
   From trauma
        Arnica   30-200
        Millefolium   30-200
        Hamamelis   30-200
   Blood, bright red
        Ipecac   30-200
        Millefolium   30-200
        Trillium   30-200
   Blood, clotted, partly fluid
        Sabina   30
        Ustilago   30
        Pulsatilla   30
   Blood, dark, clotted
        Crot.h   30
        Lachesis   30

Tereb	30
(Anthracin. as icr)	

Tubercular

Acalypha	30
Millefoliun	30
Trillium	30

With valvular disease of heart

Cactus	30
Lycopersicum	30
Hamamelis	30

Vicarious, nose, mouth, eyes (red tears)

Bryonia	30
Hamamelis	30
Phosphorus	30

HEMORRHOIDS, PILES

1.	Aloes	30
	Collinsonia	30
	Nux.vom	30
2.	Aesculus	30
	Millefolium	30
	Paeonia	30

HEMPOTYSIS *(bleeding from lungs with cough)*

Bright red blood

1.	Aconite	30
	Ferr.phos	30
	Millefolium	30
2.	Cactus	30
	Geranium	30
	Trillium	30

HEPATITIS   *See Liver, inflammation*

HODGKIN'S DISEASE *(Pseudo-leukemia)*

1.	Ars.alb	30
	Baryt.iod	30
	Scrophularia	30
2.	Ars.iod	30
	Phosphorus	30
	Acon.lyco or Acon.n	30

HYPERMETROPIA *(Far-Sightedness)*

Ruta 6x
Natrum.mur 6x
Calc. fluor 6x
(For short-sightedness see Myopia)

HYPERTENSION

With anxiety, headache, numbness and sleeplessness

Belladona 30
Ignatia 30
Coff. c 30

With palpitations, angina pectoris, sleep problems

Cactus 1x
Glonoine 1x
Passiflora 1x

With anxiety, neuroses, headaches, muscular pains and extreme depression

Aurum. met 30
Belladona 30
Rhus. tox 30

I

IMPETIGO

Antim.tart	30
Cicuta	30
Rhus.tox	30

IMPOTENCE *(also see penis, emissions, adynamia, spermatorrhoea)*

1.	Agnus. castus	30
	Caladium	30
	Selenium	30
2.	Arg.nit	30
	Conium	30
	Lycopod	30

INDIGESTION *See Dyspepsia*

INFERTILITY *See Sterility*

INFLAMMATION

1.	Aconite	30
	Belladona	30
	Bryonia	30
2.	Arnica	30
	Hep.sulph	30
	Verat.v	30

INFLUENZA *(see coryza, cough, pharyngitis, bronchitis)*

1.	Ars.alb	30
	Belladona	30
	Gelsemium	30
2.	Aconite	30
	Bryonia	30
	Cepa	30

Debility of

Chin.ars	6x
Iberis	6x
Aven.sat	6x

INGROWN TOE-NAIL *See Nails*

INJURIES *and after-effects*

	1.	Arnica	30
		Hypericum	30
		Ledum	30
	2.	Symphytum	30
		Ruta	30
		Conium	30

Bone injuries

Ruta		30
Symphytum		30
Hypericum		30
(Calc.phos as icr)		

Chronic effects of injuries

Conium	30
Nat.sulph	30
Stront.c	30

Mental symptoms, from injuries

Nat.sulph	30
Glonoine	30
Hypericum	30

Parts, rich in sentient nerves such as fingers, toes

Hypericum	30
Bellis.p	30

Surgical operation and after effects

Arnica	30
Hypericum	30
Staphysagria	30

INSANITY *(See Mania, Memory, Moods, eg. anxiety, apathetic, aversion, Delirium)*

INSECT BITES *(wasp, bee, mosquito, spider, scorpion)*

Arnica	30
Ledum	30
Apis	30

INSOMNIA   *See Sleeplessness*

INTERTRIGO *(chaffing)*   *See Erythema*

INTESTINES, INTUSSUSCEPTION, *obstruction*

	Belladona	30-200
	Merc.cor	30-200
	Plumbum	30-200

Ulceration

	Kali.bich	30
	Uran.nit	30
	Merc.cor	30

IRIS

Proplapse

	Silicea	30
	Prun.sp	30
	Kali.iod	30

IRITIS

	Aconite	30
	Euphrasia	30
	Merc.cor	30

Palstic

	Aconite	30
	Merc.cor	30
	Thuja	30

Rheumatic

	Bryonia	30
	Euphrasia	30
	Rhus.tox	30

Traumatic

	Arnica	30
	Hamamelis	30
	Ledum	30

J

JAUNDICE (*icterus*) See Liver also
Acute
1.		Card.m	30
		Bryonia	30
		Chelidonium	30
		(Phos. ac as icr)	
2.		China	30
		Mercurius	30
		Lycopod	30

Chronic
Conium	30
Phosphorus	30
Chelidonium	30

Infantile
Chamomilla	30
Merc.sol	30
Lupulus	30

JAWS
Dislocated easily
Petrolleum	30
Rhus.tox	30
Ignatia	30

Growths, swelling
Calc.fluor	30
Hekla.l	30
Thuja	30

Pain
Aconite	30
Causticum	30
Rhus.tox	30

Stiffness (trismus, lockjaw)
Cupr.met	30
Hypericum	30
Strychnine	30

JAW, LOWER

Caries, necrosis
  Phosphorus 30
  Angustura 30
  Amphisboena 30
  (Silicea as icr)

JAW, UPPER
Affections of antrum of Highmore (maxillary sinus)
  Hep.sulph 30
  Kali.iod 30
  Phosphorus 30

JOINT DISEASES   *See Rheumatism*

K

KIDNEY AFFECTIONS

ABSCESS (perinephritic)
Belladona	30
Hep.sulph	30
Merc.sol	30

ALBUMINURIA
Ars.alb	30
Kalmia	30
Merc.cor	30

ANURIA (suppression of urine: cases which need dialysis)
1.	Apis	30
	Cantharis	30
	Cupr.ars	30
2.	Lycopod	30
	Digitalis	30
	Solidago	30

INFLAMMATION (Nephritis)

Acute
1.	Apis	30
	Aur.mur	30
	Berb.vulg	30
	Cantharis	30
2.	Cupr.ars	30
	Merc.cor	30
	Tereb	30

With dropsy
Apis	6x
Apocy.c	6x
Ars.alb	6x
Helleb.n	6x
Digitalis	6x

With uraemic symptmps
Carbol.ac	6x
Chin.sulph	6x

	Hep.sulph	6x
	Merc.cor	6x

Chronic (Atrophy)

1.	Ars.alb	30
	Aur.mur	30
	Merc.cor	30
2.	Chin.sulph	30
	Digitalis	30
	Plumbum	30

KIDNEY STONES *(Renal calculi)*

General remedy

Berb.vulg	1x-6x
Hydrangea	1x-6x
Pareira. brava	1x-6x

Calcium oxalate stones: Berb.vulg Q,3x or 30
Phosphatic stones: Calc.phos or Phos.ac-3x or 6x
To eliminate the tendency

Calc.renalis	30
Calc.carb	30

RENAL COLIC

General remedies

Belladona, Berb.vulg, Cantharis, Dioscorea, Lycopod,
Nux.vom, Sarsap, Solidago, Epigea, Hydrangea

Worse, left side

Berb.vulg	1x-30
Cantharis	1x-30
Tabacum	1x-30

Worse, right side

Lycopod	30
Nux.vom	30
Ocim. can	30
Sarsaparilla	30

TUBERCULOSIS, KIDNEY   See tuberculosis

URAEMIA   *(cases which require dialysis)*

General remedies
Am.c, Belladona, Cantharis, Carbol.acid, Cupr.ars, Glonoine, Helleb, Morphing, Op, Pic.ac, Tereb, Verat.v.

URAEMIC COMA

Am. c	30
Helleb	30
Merc.cor	30
Morphine	30

URAEMIC VOMITING

Ars.iod	30
Ipecac	30

KELOID

Recent cases

Graphite	30
Sabina	30
Silicea	30

Old cases

Fluor.acid	30

(external application: Thuja-Q)

KERATITIS (*Inflammation of cornea*)

Belladona	30
Aur.mur	30
Kali.bich	30

(Merc. sol as icr)

L

LACRIMATION See Epiphora

LACTATION
Milk absent or scanty

1.	Bryonia	30
	Agnus. castus	30
2.	Agnus.c	1x-3x
3.	Phos.acid	1x-3x

Milk, excessive (Galactorrhoea): Calc.c-200, once daily or Lac.caninum-200 -1000

LABOR *(Parturition)*
Delayed
1. Caulophylum 200-1000 is specific
2. Kali. phos. 200 alternated with Caulophylum.200 after every 15 minutes.
3. If labor pains cease suddenly-Opium-200. Other remedies: Belladona, Chamomilla, China, Cimicifuga, Gelsemium, Pulsatilla

LABOR, EASY, REMEDY
1. Cauloph. 6x, three times daily during last two months of pregnancy.
2. Mag.phos 30
   Calc.phos 30
   Kali.phos 30
   Calc.fluor 30
   (dose: same as of the above formula)

LABOR
Retention of urine or Involuntary urine, after
   Causticum 200

Abdomen large, after
   Sepia 30-200
   Colocynth 30-200

LARYNGITIS
1. Aconite 30
   Ferr.phos 30
   Hep.sulph 30

2.	Belladona	30
	Causticum	30
	Merc.cor	30
	Spongia	30

LEUCODERMA *(Vitiligo)*
1. Head remedy is Ars.sul.fl. Start treatment with 3x potency, three times daily for two months. Continue the same or increase the potency according to the response.
2. Hydrocotyle, Q, 1X or 3X orally as well as applied externally.
3. Other remedies: Ars.alb, Nit.acid, Sumbul, Zinc.phos, Nat.mur
4. Old cases: Drosera, Selenium, Mang, Arg.met
5. Tuberculinum, -200-1000 as icr in all cases.
6. Look for the constitutional remedy, the similimum, any other concomitant condition and select the remedy.

LEUKAEMIA

1.	Nat. Phos	6x
	Calc.Phos	6x
	Kali.Phos	6x
	Nat. Sulph	6x
2.	Ars. Alb	6x
	Pic. Acid	6x
	Thuja	6x
	Ars.iod	6x
	(Bacil.as icr)	

LEUCOCYTOSIS

Ars. Alb	6x -30
Nat.Phos	6x -30

LEGS

Weak, difficulty in rising from a seat

Phosphorus	6x -30
Conium	6x -30
Ruta	6x -30

Coldness

Carb.Veg	30

Calc. Carb	30
Nat.mur	30
(Tabacum.as icr)	

Emaciation

Abrot	30
Kali.iod	30
Lathyrus	30

Heaviness

Alumina	30
Conium	30
Sulphur	30

Numbness, going asleep, neuropathies

Calc.Phos	6x
Causticum	6x
Cocculus	6x
(Sulpur as icr)	

Pain, in general

Bryonia	30
Gelsemium	30
Rhus.tox	30

Cramps, contractions

Cupr. ars. or (Cupr.met)	30
Lycopod	30
Rhus.tox	30

LEUCORRHOEA

1.	Calc.Phos	6x
	Kali.Phos	6x
	Kali.Sulph	6x
	Nat.Mur	6x
2.	Alumina	30
	Sepia	30
	Pulsatilla	30
	(Kreosote as icr)	

Bloody

China	30
Kreosote	30
Sepia	30

Yellow or white

Am.c	30

Pulsatilla	30
Mercurius	30

Very foetid

Kreosote	30
Carb.veg	30
Sepia	30

In Little girls

Calc.carb	6x -30
Mercurius	6x -30
Cina	6x -30

(Calc.Phos or Cubeba as icr)

Note: Calc.Phos and Sepia are specific remedies for leucorrhoea. These must be used in very case as intercurrent remedies with others.

LICHEN   *See Baker's itch*

LIPS   *See Mouth, external*

LIVER DISORDERS

ABSCESS

Belladona	30
Hep.Sulph	30
Mercurius	30

ATROPHY (Cirrhosis)

Ars.iod	30
Chelidonium	30
Phosphorus	30

CONGESTION

Aesculus	30
Aloes	30
Berb.vulg	30

CONGESTION, CHRONIC

Chelidonium	30
Choleoterinum	30
Lycopod	30

(Sulphur as icr)

ENLARGEMENT (Hypertrophy)

Ars.Alb	30
Chelidionum	30

Chionanthus	30

INFLAMMATION, Hepatitis (all types)

Bryonia	30
Chelidonium	30
Ceanothus	30

CANCER

Cholesterinum	30
Chelidonium	30
Phosphorus	30

CIRRHOSIS WITH ASCITES

Lycopod	30
Ars.Alb	30
Phosphorus	30

LICE

Sulphur	30
Staphysagria	30
Lycopod	30

(For external use, Staphysagria-Q, half teaspoon mixed in four teaspoons of coconut oil or soft yellow paraffin, once daily).

LIPOMA

1.	Baryt.carb	6x
	Phytolacca	6x
2.	Lapis alb	6x
	Uric.ac	6x

(For external application use Thuja-Q, twice daily).

LOCOMOTOR ATAXIA

1.	Head Remedies are Anagalus and Alumina	
2.	Plumbum	6x
	Arg.nit	6x
	Alumina	6x
3.	Start treatment with Bacilinum-200. Also use Strych.sul-200 or Atropin.sul-200 as icr	

LUMBAGO   *See Backache*

LUNGS

Abscess

Belladona	30
Hep.sulph	30

Silicea 30

Congestion
Aconite 6x
Ferr.Phos 6x
Belladona 6x

Congestion, Passive
Carb.veg 30
Digitalis 30
Sulphur 30

Infiltration with eosinophils
1. Ars.Alb-200 once daily for few days; if no change occurs then use following formula.
2. Ars.Alb 30
Spongia 30
Iodum 30
(Drosera as icr)

Oedema (Pulmonary oedema)
Am. carb 6x
Phosphorus 6x
Sanguinaria 6x
(Tub. as icr)

M

MALARIA
Recent cases
	Chin.sulph	30
	Nat.mur	30
	Ars.alb	30

Periodical, every week, month or year
	Ars.alb	30
	China	30
	Eupator.perf	30

Prophylactic for malaria
1. Malaria of-200, twice in a month.
2. Chin.sul-30, twice weekly during malaria season.

MAMMARY GLANDS, AFFECTIONS
CANCER
1. Conium — 30
   Calc.fluor — 30
   Slicea — 30
2. Other remedies: Arg.nit, Ars.alb, Aster.rub, Card.m, Condurango, Carcinosin, Conium, Galium, Hydrastis, Kal.iod, Plumb.iod, Scirrhinum, Thuja.

INDURATION, HARDNESS
1. Phytolacca — 6x
   Conium — 6x
2. Bryonia — 6x
   Calc.fluor — 6x
   (Asterias rub. 200 or 1000 as icr)

INFLAMMTION (Mastitis)
1. Belladona — 30
   Bryonia — 30
2. Conium — 30
   Phytolacca — 30
   (Lac.can.200 as icr)

NIPPLES, CRACKS, FISSURES, SORE
Arnica — 30
Graphite — 30
Phytolacca — 30

MANIA

1.	Stramon	30-200
	Belladona	30-200
	Hyoscyamus	30-200
	(Tarent.H,200 as icr)	
2.	Anacard	30-200
	Cimicifuga	30-200
	Elaterium	30-200

MARASMUS *(Emaciation, atrophy, malnutrition)*

1.	Abrot	6X
	Nat.mur	6X
	Iodum	
2.	Ars.alb	6X
	Calc.carb	6X
	Lycopod	6X
3.	Abrot	6x
	Iodum	6x
	Oleum.jecoris	6x

MASTOID DISEASES
1. Head remedies: Capsicum and Hep.sulph
2. Inflammation (Mastoiditis)

Aur.met	30
Capsicum	30
Nit.acid	30

MASTURBATION, *ill-effects*

Conium	30
Lycopod	30
Staphysagria	30

MEASLES
With cough, ear or joint pains

Bryonia	6x
Kali.bich	6x
Plusatilla	6x
(Sticta as icr)	

With eye symptoms predominant

Belladona	6x
Ars.alb	6x
Gelsemium	6x
Euphrasia	6x

With cerebral and convulsive symptoms

Belladona	30

	Cupr.met	30
	Zinc.met	30

With rash, retrocedent, or slow development

	Bryonia	6x
	Cupr.met	6x
	Zinc.met	6x
	(Stram.as icr)	

MIGRAINE

1.		Belladona	30
		Coff.c	30
2.		Iris.v	30
		Sanguinaria	30

Left half

	Onosmod	30
	Spigelia	30
	Nat.mur	30
	(Nux.vom as icr)	

Right half

	Sanguinaria	30
	Chelidonium	30
	Kali.bich	30
	(Iris.v as icr)	

MEMORY

Head remedies: Anacard, Baryt.c Kali.phos. Nux.vom. Weak or lost(cannot remember familiar streets, right words (amnesic aphasia, paraphasia). Thoughts vanish while reading, talking, writing.

	Anacard	6x
	Lycopod	6x
	Sulphur	6x

Difficulty of fixing attention

	Gelsemium	6x
	Nux.vom	6x
	Aethusa	6x

Omits letters or words

	Kali.brom	6x
	Nux.mos	6x
	Lycopod	6x

MENOPAUSE   *See Climacteric*

MENSTRUATION DISORDERS
Amenorrhoea

1.	Plusatilla	30-200
	Ferr.phos	30-200
	Kali.phos	30-200
2.	Pulsatilla	30-200
	Dulcamara	30-200
	Senecio	30-200
	(Tub.as icr)	

MENSTRUATION
Before the proper age

Calc.carb	30
Sabina	30
Carb.veg	30

Delayed first menses

Graphite	30
Kali.carb	30
Senecio	30
(Puls.200 as icr)	

Dysmenorrhoea (Painful menses) See Dysmenorrhoea
Menorrhagia (excessive menstrual flow)
After miscarriage, labor

Cimicifuga	30
Sabina	30
Ustilago	30
(Nit.acid as icr)	

Before expected date

Millefolium	30
Trillium	30
Thlaspi	30

MENSTRUATION
Complaints, preceding and during flow
  Abdomen distended.

China	30
Kreosote	30
Nux.vom	30

  Breasts, tender, swollen

Conium	30

Helonias	30
Phytolacca	30

Headache

Belladona	30
Gelsemium	30
Nat.mur	30

Hysterical symptoms

Cimicifuga	30
Ignatia	30
Mag.mur	30

Mania

Cimicifuga	30
Dulcamara	30
Stramon	30

Pain labor like, extending down hip, to groins, thighs and legs

Caulophylum	30
Gelsemium	30
Sepia	30

Pain in ovaries

Apis	30
Cimicifuga	30
Lachesis	30

METRITIS, ENDOMETRITIS

Acute

Ars.alb	30
Cimicifuga	30
Sepia	30

Chronic

Aur.m. n	30
Calc.carb	30
Sabina	30
(Ars.alb, 200 as icr)	

Haemorrhagic cases

Hamamelis	30
Thlaspi	30
Secal.cor	30

MENIERE'S DISEASE *(also see Vertigo)*
    Chenopod   30
    Chin.sulph   30
    Nat.sulph   30
Others: Baryt.mur, Chin.sul, Tabac, Therid.

MENINGITIS
1. Apis   30
   Bryonia   30
   Cicuta   30
2. Cupr.met   30
   Belladona   30
   Gelsemium   30
3. Cupr.ars   30
   Helleb   30
   Zinc.met   30

Others: Op. Sil, Sulphur.Tuberculinum

Tubercular
    Calc.Phos   30
    Helleb   30
    Iodof   30
    (Bacil. as icr)

METRORRHAGIA
General formula
    Hamamelis   30-200
    Ipecac   30-200
    Trillium   30-200
From fibroids
    Phosphorus   30-200
    Thlaspi   30-200

MOODS, PSYCHIATRIC DISORDERS
Anxiety
    Pulsatilla   30
    Ignatia   30
    Nux.vom   30
    (Calc.carb as icr)
Apathetic, indifferent to everything
    Gelsemium   30

| | | Ignatia | 30 |
| | | Sepia | 30 |

Aversion to physical and mental work, indecisive

1.	Aloe	30
	Ignatia	30
	Sulphur	30
2.	Baryt.carb	30
	Kali.phos	30
	Carb.veg	30

MORNING SICKNESS *See Pregnancy*

MORPHINE (Opium) ADDICTION
Eating habit and ill-effects

1.	Verat.alb	30-200
	Nux.vom	30-200
	Ars.alb	30-200
2.	Avena sativa-Q, 20 drops four times daily, in warm water.	

Smoking habit (Heroin addiction)

| Avena sativa-Q | 10-20 drops |
| Passiflora -Q | 10-20 drops |

(three or four times daily, in warm water)

MORTIFICATION *from an offence See Aggravation*

MOUTH, INNER *(buccal cavity)*

Bleeding, after tooth extraction

Phosphorus	30
Nat.mur	30
Arnica	30

Canker-sores

Borax	30
Merc.cor	30
Nit.acid	30

Dryness

Ars.alb	30
Bryonia	30
Lycopod	30

Glands, salivary, inflamed

Hep.sulph	30
Merc.sol	30
Mur.acid	30

Inflammation (Stomatitis)
- Merc.sol — 30
- Borax — 30
- Nit.acid — 30

Inflammation.aphthous(Thrush)
- Borax — 30
- Merc.sol — 30
- Sulphur — 30

Inflammation, ulcerative
- Ars.alb — 30
- Merc.sol — 30
- Hep.sulph — 30

Pain in mouth, from plate of teeth
- Alumen — 30
- Borax — 30

MOUTH, EXTERNAL

Corners, pearly white color
- Cina — 6x
- Aethusa — 6x
- Santonin — 6x

Cracks, ulcerations
- Antim.crud — 6x
- Hep.sulph — 6x
- Nit.acid — 6x

Eruptions, around
- Ars.alb — 6x
- Graphite — 6x
- Nat.mur — 6x

MOUTH, LIPS

Black, cyanosed
- Ars.alb — 6x
- Merc.cor — 6x
- Bryonia — 6x
- (Vipera as icr)

Blue, cyanosed
- Cupr.met — 6x
- Verat.alb — 6x
- Carb.veg — 6x

Cracks, ulcer in middle of lower lip
Kali.mur	6x
Nat.mur	6x
Hep.sulph	6x

Dryness
Bryonia	6x
Nat.mur	6x

Numbness, tingling
Aconite	6x
Nat.mur	6x
Echinacea	6x

Picks them untill they bleed
Arum.tri	6x
Zinc.met	6x
Helleb	6x

Swelling of lower lip
Pulsatilla	30
Sepia	30
Kali.sulph	30

Swelling of upper lip
Hep.sulph	30
Apis	30
Calc.phos	30

MUMPS *(Parotitis)*

1.	Belladona	30
	Merc.cor	30
	Pulsatilla	30
2.	Clematis	30
	Ferr.phos	30
	Kali.bich	30

With metastases to testes
Clematis	30
Pulsatilla	30
Hamamelis	30

Muscae volitantes *(spots before eyes) See optical illusions*

MUSCLES
INFLAMMATION (MYOSITIS) AND PAIN
Arnica	30
Hypericum	30
Rhus.tox	30

PAIN (Myalgia)
Arnica	30
Bryonia	30
Cimicifuga	30
(Rhus.tox as icr)	

SORENESS
Arnica	30
Baptisia	30
Rhus.tox	30

WEAKNESS, DEBILITY
Conium	30
Gelsemium	30
Kali.phos	30

MYELITIS (inflammation of spinal cord)
Acute
Ars.alb	6x
Oxal.acid	6x
Nux.vom	6x
(Phos. as icr)	

Chronic
Plumb.met	30
Zinc.phos	30
Strychnine	30
(Lathyrus as icr)	

MYOPIA (short-sightedness)
Agaricus.m	6x
Gelsemium	6x
Physostigma	6x

MYXOEDEMA (Hypothyroidism)
Prim.ob	6x
Thyroidin	6x
Pituitrin.	6x
(Ars.alb as icr)	

NAILS, AFFECTIONS

General remedies Ant.c, Graph.Sil, Alumina, Hyperic, Nit.ac, Upas, X-ray, Dioscorea

ATROPHY   Silicea
BITING OF   Am.brom, Arum.tri
BLUENESS Digitalis   (see cyanosis)

DEFORMED, brittle, thick

Antim.c	6x
Ars.alb	6x
Graphite	6x
(Silicea as icr)	

ERUPTIONS, around

Graphite	30
Stan.mur	30
(Psorin.as icr)	

FALLING OFF

Dioscorea	30
Butyr.ac	30
Helleborus	30

INFLAMMATION

1.	Dioscorea	30
	Hep.sulph	30
2.	Nat.sulph	30
	Calc.sulph	30

INFLAMMATION, of pulp (Onychia)

Fluor.ac	30
Graphite	30
Silicea	30

INGROWING TOE NAIL (Magnet.Australis is specific remedy)

Graphite	30
Silicea	30
Nit.acid	30

INJURY, to matrix   Hypericum   30-200

SKIN AROUND, dry, cracked
1. Graphite 6x
   Nat.mur 6x
2. Petroleum 6x
   Kali.mur 6x

SPOTS, white on
Alumina 6x
Nit.acid 6x

NAUSEA
1. Specific remedy Ipecac 30-200
2. Ipecac 30
   Carb.veg 30
   Ars.alb 30
3. Bryonia 30
   Nux.vom 30
   Pulsatilla 30

NECROSIS
Long Bones
Asafoetida 30
Mezerium 30
Stront.c 30

Vertebrae
Calc.carb 30
Nat.mur 30
Phos.acid 30

NEPHRITIS *See Kidney*
NEPHROLITHIASIS *See Kidney stones*
NEURALGIA
Brachial plexus, cervico-brachial, cervical spondylosis
Rhus.tox 30
Kalmia 30
Sulphur 30

Ciliary (ciliary neuralgia with or without glaucoma)
Cinnabaris 6x

	Gelsemium	6x
	Cimicifuga	6x

Face (trigeminal neuralgia and others)
1.		Aconite	30
		Ars.alb	30
2.		Belladona	30
		Chamomilla	30

Reflex, from decayed teeth
	Mezerium	30
	Merc.sol	30
	Staphysagria	30

Unilateral, left
1.		Aconite	30
		Colocynthis	30
2.		Pulsatilla	30
		Mag.phos	30

Intercostal, with cough
1.		Chelidonium	30
		Bryonia	30
2.		Cimicifuga	30
		Ranun.b	30

Sciatica   *See Sciatica*

Spermatic cord
	Colocynthis	30
	Cantharis	30
	Belladona	30

Uterine
	Cimicifuga	30
	Sepia	30
	Colocynthis	30

NEURASTHENIA *(nervous prostration)*

See Adynamia also

General remedies: Anac, Aven.s, Calc.ph, China, Coccul, Gels, Kali.ph, Nux.v, Phos, Phos.ac, Zinc.m

Unable to apply mind, weak memory
Anacard	30

	Gelsemium	30
	Kali.phos	30

From long continued grief
	Ignatia	30
	Phos.acid	30
	Nux.vom	30

Hypochondriacal tendency
	Aur.met	6x
	Nat.mur	6x
	Podophyllum	6x
	(Sulphur as icr)	

Sexual origin
	Agnus.castus	6x
	Staphysagria	6x
	Caladium	6x

NEURITIS (*inflammation of the nerves*)

General formula
	Nux.vom	6x
	Strychnin	6x
	Hypericum	6x
	Cepa	6x

In legs (anterior crural, circumflex, lesser sciatic nerves)
	Kalmia	6x
	Sanguinaria	6x
	Aesculus	6x

Retrobulbar, with sudden loss of sight
	Arg.nit	6x
	Nat.mur	6x
	Phosphorus	6x

NIGHT-TERRORS

1.		Chamomilla	6x
		Belladona	6x
2.		Cina	6x
		Calc.carb	6x

NIPPLES

Cracks, fissures, ulcers, inflamed, sore
	Arnica	6x
	Graphite	6x

Nit.acid	6x

Nodes, lymphatic, inflamed, enlarged

Badiaga	30
Merc.sol	30
Hep.sulph	30
(Conium-200 as icr)	

NODOSITIES, TOPHI *(due to gout or arthritis)*

Am. phos	6x
Lycopod	6x
Caulophyllum	6x

NOSE, *CARIES, periostitis, ulcer*

Hekla.l	6x
Aur.met	6x
Kali.bich	6x
(Hep.sulph-200 as icr)	

NOSE, EXTERNAL

FRACKLES

Sepia	6x
Phosphorus	6x
Sulphur	6x

FURUNCLES

Hep.sulph	30
Sepia	30
Nat.mur	30

PUSTULES

Hap.sulph	30
Silicea	30
Calc.sulph	30

WARTS

Causticum	30
Thuja	30

ECZEMA (alae-wings of nose)

Mezerium	6x
Petroleum	6x
Graphite	6x

NOSE, INTERNAL

ABSCESS, of septum; boil inside

Belladona	30

Hep.sulph		30
Aconite		30

EPISTAXIS

Millefolium		6x
Ferr.phos		6x
Carb.veg		6x
(Hamamelis. 200)		

With menses absent (vicarious)

Bryonia		6x
Hamamelis		6x
Phosphorus		6x

With trauma, operations

Arnica		30
Hamamelis		30
Thlaspi		30

NOSE

BLOWING, boring, digging into

1.	Hydrastis	30
	Sticta	30
2.	Arum.tri	30
	Cina	30

CONGESTION, violent type

1.	Melilotus	30
	Belladona	30
2.	Cupr.m	30
	Lemna.m	30

NASAL DRYNESS

1.	Nux.moschata-30 is the remedy of choice	
2.	Sticta	30
	Aconite	30
3.	Lycopod	30
	Sulphur	30

POLYPI

Phosphorus		30
Sanguinaria		30
Lemna.m		30

RHINOSCLEROMA (hardness)

Calc.fluor		6x

Aur.m. n	6x
Conium	6x

NOSTALGIA *(home-sickness)*
Capsicum	6x
Ignatia	6x
Phos.ac	6x

NYMPHOMANIA
Cantharis	30
Phosphorus	30
Murex	30

O

OBESITY *(adiposis, corpulence)*

	1.	Calc.carb	6x
		Fucus.v	6x
		Thyroid	6x
	2.	Calc.carb	6x
		Capsicum	6x
		Ferr.met	6x

OEDEMA *(dropsy)*

From heart disease

Apis		6x
Digitalis		6x
Merc.cor		6x

From liver disease

1.	Bryonia		6x
	Card.m		6x
2.	Lycopod		6x
	Chelidonium		6x

Abdomen (Ascites)

Ars.alb	6x
Lycopod	6x
China	6x

Chest (Hydrothorax)

Digitalis	6x
Kali.c	6x
Merc.sol	6x
(Sulphur.as.icr)	

OESOPHAGUS

Burning, smarting

Iris.v	30
Cantharis	30
Merc.cor	30

Constriction, dysphagia

Belladona	30
Asafoetida	30
Gelsemium	30

OLD AGE, *effects of; See Senile decay, Dementia, Adynamia*

OPHTHALMIA

Catarrhal, purulent
Euphrasia	30
Belladona	30
Merc.sol	30

Neonatorum
Arg.nit	6x
Hep.sulph	6x
Merc.cor	6x

OPTIC NERVE

Atrophy
1.	Phosphorus	30
	Strych.n	30
2.	Nux.vom	30
	Tabacum	30

Inflammation
Ars.alb	30
Merc.cor	30
Nux.vom	30

OPTICAL ILLUSIONS

Flashes, flames, stars
1.	Belladona	30
	Cyclamen	30
2.	Physostigma	30
	Nat.mur	30

Halo around light
Sulphur	30
Hyoscyamus	30
Belladona	30

Spots (muscae volitantes)
China	30
Merc.cor	30
Nux.vom	30

(Phos. as icr)

OSTEOMYELITIS *(infection of bone marrow)*
Chin.sulph	30
Phosphorus	30
Calc.phos	30

OTITIS MEDIA *(middle ear inflammation)*

Catarrhal, acute
Belladona	30
Hep.sulph	30
Merc.sol	30

Suppurative, acute (with mastoiditis)
Capsicum	30
Hep.sulph	30
Merc.sol	30

Suppurative, chronic
Hep.sulph	30
Kali.bich	30
Merc.sol	30

OTORRHOEA *(ear discharge)*

Bloody discharge
Hep.sulph	30
Merc.sol	30
Ars.alb	30

Foetid, acrid or bland
1.	Calc.sulph	30
	Kali, sulph	30
2.	Silicea	30
	Ferr.phos	30

OTALGIA *(pain in ear)*
Ferr.phos	30
Mag.phos	30
Belladona	30

Pulsating, throbbing
1.	Belladona	30
	Ferr.phos	30

2.	Glonoine		30
	Merc.sol		30

OVARIES, DISEASES OF
Atrophy
Iodum	30
Oophorinum	30
Orchitinum	30
Staphysagria	30

Cysts, dropsy
Apis	6x
Aur.iod	6x
Colocynth	6x
Oophorinum	6x

Inflammation (Oophoritis)
Acute
1.	Apis	30
	Colocynth	30
2.	Merc.cor	30
	Pulsatilla	30

Chronic
Conium	30
Iodum	30
Thuja	30

Pain *(Ovaralgia)*
General remedy
Apis	30
Colocynth	30
Staphysagria	30

Left ovary
Arg.met	30
Lachesis	30
Colocynthis	30

Right ovary
Bryonia	30
Lycopod	30

Podophyllum	30
Ovaries, *Removal, after effects of*	
Colocynthis	30
Oophorinum	30
Orchitinum	30
Staphysagria	30

P

PALATE

Red, swollon
Apis	30
Aur.met	30
Merc.cor	30

Ulceration, rawness
Arum.tri	30
Nit.ac	30
Merc.cor	30

PALPITATION See Heart

PANARITIUM *(felon, whitlow of finger-nails)*
See also Nail inflammation

Treatment and Prevention
Dioscorea	30
Hep.sulph	30
Merc.sol	30

PANCREAS, AFFECTIONS
Iris.v	30
Merc.sol	30
Ars.alb	30

PARALYSIS *(also see gait disorders)*

Agitans (Parkinsonism)
Aur.m	30-200
Conium	30-200
Plumbum	30-200

Hemiplegia, left
1.	Arnica		30-200
	Belladona		30-200
2.	Lachesis		30-200
	Cocculus		30-200

Hemiplegia, right
1.	Causticum		30-200

2.	Belladona	30-200
	Lycopod	30-200
	Iridium	30-200

Infantile (Poliomyelitis)
Causticum	30-200
Gelsemium	30-200
Plumbum	30-200

Paraplegia
Arg.nit	30
Conium	30
Gelsemium	30

Pneumogastric (of lungs)
Antim.tart	30
Ipecac	30
Lauroc	30
Ars.alb	30

Forearm (Wrist-drop)
Plumbum	30-200
Ruta	30-200
Silicea	30-200

Sphinctres
Causticum	30-200
Gelsemium	30-200
Phosphorus	30-200

Throat, vocal cords
Causticum	30-200
Gelsemium	30-200
Bothrops.1	30-200

PAROTITIS *(Mumps)*
Pulsatilla	30
Merc.sol	30
Belladona	30

Metastases to mammae, ovaries, testes
Conium	30
Clematis	30
Pulsatilla	30

PELVIC AFFECTIONS

Abscess

Hep.sulph	30-200
Merc.sol	30-200
Silicea	30-200

Peritonitis

Apis	30-200
Hep.sulph	30-200
Merc.sol	30-200
Silicea	30-200

PEMPHIGUS

Ars.alb	30
Cantharis	30
Rhus.tox	30

PENIS, AFFECTIONS

Atrophy, small in size

Agnus.castus	30
Arg.m	30
Staphysagria	30

Priapism (painful erections) See Chordee

Pustules

Ars.alb	30
Hep.sulph	30
Merc.sol	30

Rash and spots

Sulphur	30
Rhus.tox	30
Merc.sol	30

Swollen, inflamed glans

Apis	30
Cantharis	30
Merc.sol	30

Warts, condylomata (all types)

Cinnaberis	30
Nit.acid	30
Causticum	30
Thuja	30

PERICARDITIS *See Heart*

PERIOSTITIS, *and periosteal affections See Bones*

PERITONITIS
Acute
Bryonia	30-200
Merc.sol	30-200
Copaiva	30-200

Chronic
Lycopod	30-200
Merc.cor	30-200
Sulphur	30-200

PERTUSSIS *(Whooping cough)*
Drosera	30
Cupr.met	30
Ipecac	30

PETECHIAE *(subcutaneous bleeding spots)*
Arnica	30
Sul.acid	30
Phosphorus	30

PHTHRIASIS *(lice)*
Nat.mur	30
Sabadila	30
Staphysagria	30

(Sabad.Q as shampo and Psorin.or Bacil.as icr)

PETIT MAL EPILEPSY *See Epilepsy*

PHARYNGITIS *(inflammation, atrophic, sicca)*
Alumina	30
Kali.bich	30
Nux.vom	30

Catarrhal, acute or chronic
Belladona	30
Hep.sul	30

Merc.sol	30
Baryt.carb	30

PHLEBITIS *(inflammation of veins)*
Hamamelis	30
Ars.alb	30
Apis	30

PHLEGMASIA ALBA DOLENS *(Milk-leg)*
Ars.alb	30-200
Rhus.tox	30-200
Hamamelis	30-200

PHOBIAS *(Fears)*

Of crowds, crossing streets
Aconite	30-200
Platina	30-200

Of people (Anthropophobia)
Aconite.n	30
Staphysagria	30
Aur.met	30

Solitude
Gelsemium	30
Lycopod	30
Pulsatilla	30

Stage-fright
Gelsemium	30
Anacard	30
Arg.nit	30

PHOSPHATURIA   *See Urine*

PHOTOPHOBIA
Belladona	30
Euphrasia	30
Merc.sol	30

PHTHISIS, *pulmonalis*   *See Tuberculosis*
PICA *(morbid appetite) See Appetite*
PITYRIASIS *(dermatitis exfoliativa)*

Ars.alb	30
Mezerium	30
Sulphur	30

PILES   *See Hemorrhoids*

PLEURISY

Merc.sol	30
Ranun.b	30
Sulphur	30

With adhesions

Hep.sulph	30
Ranun.b	30
Sulphur	30

With tuberculosis

Bryonia	30
Iodum	30
Hep.sulph	30

PNEUMONIA *(Broncho-pneumonia)*

Ipecac	30
Bryonia	30
Ferr.phos	30
Chelidonium	30

POISONING *(decayed food)*

Cupr.ars	30
Carb.veg	30
Pulsatilla	30

POLIOMYELITIS   *See Paralysis*

POLYCHROME SPECTRA, optical *illusions*

Black before eyes

Belladona	30
Carb.veg	30
Tabacum	30

Flashes, flames, flickering

Belladona	30
Cyclamen	30
Iris.v	30

Sparks, stars

Belladona		30
Cyclamen		30
Glonoine		30

Spots (muscae volitantes)

Merc.sol		30
China		30
Phosphorus		30

POLYPS

All types

Calc.carb		30
Phosphorus		30
Lemna.m		30
(Thuja.200 as icr)		

Nose

Calc.phos		30
Kali.sulph		30
Ferr.phos		30
Silicea		30

Uterus, fibroids, polyps

Aur.mur		30
Calc.iod		30
Conium		30
Thuja		30

POLYURIA *(copious, profuse urine output)*

Ignatia		30
Nat.mur		30
Equisatum		30

PORTAL CONGESTION

Aloes		30
Collinsonia		30
Sulphur		30

POST-NASAL DISEASES *(naso-pharynx)*

Inflammation, acute

Aconite		30
Kali.bich		30
Merc.cor		30

Inflammation, chronic

Hydrastis	30
Merc.cor	30
Spigelia	30

Inflammation, chronic, with post-nasal dropping

Alumina	30
Kali.bich	30
Spigelia	30

PREGNANCY, DISORDERS

ALBUMINURIA
Apis	30
Cupr.ars	30
Merc.cor	30

BACKACHE
Aesculus	30
Kali.c	30

BREASTS, PAINFUL
Belladona	30
Bryonia	30

CONSTIPATION - *(Nux.v-30 is the head remedy)*
Collinsonia	30
Platina	30
Sepia	30

COUGH
Nux.vom	30
Bryonia	30
Causticum	30

CRAMPS, IN CALVES
Cupr.met	30
Mag.phos	30
Nux.vom	30

CRAVING, ABNORMAL   *See Appetite*

DIARRHOEA *(head remedy - Puls. 30, four hourly)*
Pulsatilla	30
Ferr.met	30
Sulphur	30

MORNING SICKNESS *(nausea, vomiting)*
Ipecac	30

Symphoricarpus	30
Ars.alb	30

OEDEMA
Ars.alb	6x
Ferr.phos	6x
Sulphur	6x

PAINFUL, MOVEMENT OF FETUS
Pulsatilla	30
Thuja	30

PALPITATION
Cactus	3x-30
Belladona	3x-30
Nux.vom	3x-30

PRURITUS, VULVA AND VAGINA
Caladium	30
Sepia	30
Collinsonia	30

SALIVATION
Jaborandi	30
Merc.sol	30
Nat.mur	30

SEXUAL EXCITEMENT-See Nymphomania also
Head remedy is Platina	30

SLEEPLESSNESS
Coff.c	30
Nux.vom	30
Sulphur	30

TOOTHACHE
Calc.fluor	30
Kreosotum	30
Staphysagria	30
Merc.sol	30

TOXAEMIC CONDITIONS: *Head remedy is Kali.mur,*
30-200

URINE, FREQUENCY
Causticum	30
Belladona	30

Nux.vom	30

VARICOSE VEINS
Carb.veg	30
Hamamelis	30
Arnica	30

VERTIGO
Cocculus	30
Nux.vom	30
Belladona	30

PPRIAPISM *See Chordee*
PROCTITIS
Aloes	30
Collinsonia	30
Merc.cor	30

PROLAPSUS ANI
Podophyllum	30
Ruta	30
Ignatia	30

PROLAPSUS, UTERI *(displacement)*
Alet, far	30
Calc.carb	30
Helonias	30

PROLAPSUS, VAGINAE
Lappa	30
Sepia	30
Kreosotum	30

PROSOPALGIA *(face-ache, neuralgia)* See Neuralgia
PROSTATE GLAND

General remedy
Ferr.pic	30
Sabal.s	30
Thuja	30

Hypertrophy
Chimaphila	30
Baryt.carb	30
Sulphur	30

PROSTATE, Inflammation (prostatitis)

Acute

Chimaphila	30
Merc.d	30
Staphysagria	30

Chronic

Aur.met	30
Conium	30
Merc.cor	30
(Selen.as icr)	

PRURITUS, DERMATITIS, ECZEMA

General remedy

Ars.alb	30
Lycopod	30
Sulphur	30

Of genitals

Ambra.grisea	6x
Caladium	6x
Sepia	6x

Of webs of fingers, bends of joints

Hep.sulph	6x
Selenium	6x
Sepia	6x

Amelioration from cold

Graphite	6x
Mezerium	6x
Berb.vulg	6x

Amelioration from warmth

Ars.alb	30
Petroleum	30

Worse from undressing, warmth of bed

Alumina	6x
Ars.alb	6x
Nat.sulph	6x

PSORIASIS

Ars.alb	30

Lycopod	30
Sulphur	30

PTERYGIUM (*a triangular patch of mucous membrane growing on the conjunctiva usually on the nasal side of the eye*)

Can.sat	30
Sulphur	30
Zinc.met	30

PTYALISM (*salivation*)

Merc.sol	30
Nit.acid	30
Iris.v	30

PULMONARY OEDEMA

Antim.tart	30
Ars.alb	30
Kali.c	30

PUERPERIUM (*lying-in period*)

Pains, lower abdomen, groins, shins

Cupr.met	30
Carb.veg	30
Caulophyllum	30

Haemorrhage

Hamamelis	6x
China	6x
Sabina	6x
Secale.cor	6x

Haemorrhoids

Aloes	30
Ignatia	30
Pulsatilla	30

Lochia, acrid, bloody; scanty or offensive

Kreosotum	30
Nit.acid	30
Secale.cor	30

Fever (milk-fever)

Baptisia	30-200
Chin.sulph	30-200

	Rhus.tox	30-200
	(Pyrogen-200 as icr)	
Mania		
	Can.ind	30-200
	Hyoscyamus	30-200
	Stramonium	30-200

PULSE

Full, round, bounding, strong, felt all over
- Belladona — 30
- Glonoine — 30
- Cactus — 30

Intermittent
- Cratagus — 30
- Carb.veg — 30
- Nat.mur — 30

Irregular
- Ars.alb — 30
- Aur.met — 30
- Cactus — 30

Rapid (tachycardia)
- Belladona — 6x
- Cactus — 6x
- Gelsemium — 6x
- Carb.veg — 6x

PUPILS, *Contracted (miosis)*
- Physostigma — 30
- Opium — 30
- Gelsemium — 30

Dilated (mydriasis)
- Belladona — 30
- Cicuta — 30
- Stramonium — 30

PURPURA
- Arnica — 30
- Hamamelis — 30
- Sulph.ac — 30

PYELITIS *(inflammation of pelvis of kidney)*

Acute
Ars.alb	6x
Belladona	6x
Carb.veg	6x
Merc.cor	6x

Calculous
Hydrangea	30
Lycopod	30
Uva.u	30

Chronic
Cppaiva	6x
Chimaphila	6x
Berb.vulg	6x
Juniparus	6x

PYEMIA, septicemia

Arnica	30
Chin.ars	30
Echinacea	30

PYLORUS

Constriction
China	6x
Nux.vom	6x
Phosphorus	6x

Pain
Hep.sulph	30
Lycopod	30
Uran.n	30

PYORRHOEA, ALVEOLARIS

Merc.sol	30
Staphysagria	30
Silicea	30

PYROSIS *(heartburn)*

Calc.carb	6x
Bismuth	6x
Ars.alb	6x

        Carb.veg   6x

PYURIA *(pus in urine)*
Benz.ac	30
Ars.alb	30
Cantharis	30

R

RECTUM

ABSCESS (Peri-rectal)
Sulphur	30
Aloes	30
Cantharis	30
Capsicum	30

BURNING
Ars.alb	30
Ratanhia	30
Sulphur	30
Nit.acid	30

PARETIC conditions
Causticum	30
Gelsemium	30
Aloes	30
Phosphorus	30

RENAL COLIC *See Kidney Stones*
Berb.vulg	30
Cantharis	30
Sarsaparilla	30
Lycopod	30

RETINA

Apoplexy(haemorrhage)
Arnica	30
Crotal.h	30
Hamamelis	30

Congestion
Belladona	30
Aur.met	30
Ferr.phos	30

Detachment
Aur.mur	30
Gelsemium	30
Naphthaline	30

Injury

Arnica	30
Hamamelis	30
Ledum	30

Thrombosis and degeneration

Hamamelis	30
Phosphorus	30
Belladona	30

RHEUMATISM, *Arthritis, Joints*

Articular

Bryonia	30
Rhus.tox	30
Ferr.phos	30

Joints, large

Rhus.tox	30
Bryonia	30
Merc.sol	30

Joints, small

Caulophyllum	30
Ledum	30
Sabina	30

RHEUMATISM, *CHRONIC*

Am. phos	30
Causticum	30
Rhus.tox	30

RHINITIS

Acute (Cold in head), Hay fever, Summer catarrh

Sabadilla	30
Nat.mur	30
Ars.alb	30

Predisposition to

Calc.carb	30
Hep.sulph	30
Nat.mur	30

Coryza, worse in warm room, better in open air

Ars.alb	30
Nux.vom	30
Cepa	30

Coryza, with lachrymation, sneezing

Ars.alb	30
Justicia	30
Euphrasia	30
Nat.mur	30

Coryza, purulant esp in children

Kali.bich	30
Hep.sulph	30
Calc.carb	30

RICKETS

Calc.phos	30
Ferr.phos	30
Silicea	30

RINGWORM *(Trichophytosis)*

Graphite	30
Sepia	30
Tellurium	30

RUBELLA *(German measles)*

Ars.alb	30
Merc.cor	30
Euphrasia	30

S

SALPINGITIS *(inflammation of fallopian tubes)*
Colocynth	30
Merc.cor	30
Ars.alb	30

SCABIES
Sulphur	30
Merc.sol	30
Hep.sulph	30

SCALP AFFECTIONS
Dandruff(seborrhoea)
Ars.alb	30
Bryonia	30
Sulphur	30

SCALP, Eruptions
Boils
Hep.sulph	30
Calc.sulph	30
Antim.tart	30

Crusta lactea
Vinca min	30
Hep.sulph	30
Mezereum	30

Eczema
Calc.carb	30
Graphite	30
Petroleum	30

Growths, tumors, exostoses
Calc.fluor	30
Kali.iod	30
Mercurius	30

Moist, humid eruptions
Calc.carb	30
Rhus.tox	30

Mezereum		30

Pustules

Clematis		30
Mezereum		30
Graphite		30

Ringworm (Tinea capitis), alopecia

Tellurium		6x
Mezereum		6x
Graphite		6x

Itching

Bovista		6x
Sulphur		6x
Ars.alb		6x

Numbness

Petroleum		6x
Aconite		6x
Alumina		6x

Sensitive, to touch, combing

Belladona		6x
China		6x
Gelsemium		6x

Sweat, excessive

Calc.carb		30
Silicea		30
Calc.phos		30

SCIATICA

1.	Rhus.tox		30
	Colocynthis		30
	Gnaphalium		30
2.	Sulphur		30
	Bryonia		30
	Aconite		30
3.	Chamomilla		30
	Ignatia		30

In Rheumatic cases

1.	Bryonia		30
	Cimicifuga		30
	Guaiacum		30
2.	Ledum		30
	Rhus.tox		30

		Kalmia	30

SCLERODERMA *(hide bound skin)*
	1.	Thyroidin	30
		Bryonia	30
	2.	Hydrocotyle	30
		Ars.alb	30

SCLERITIS *(inflammation of sclera of eye)*
	1.	Ars.alb	30
		Merc.cor	30
	2.	Hep.sulph	30
		Spigelia	30

SCROFULOUS DISEASES
Ars.iod	30
Baryt.carb	30
Ferr.phos	30

SCROTUM, *Eczema*
Graphite	6x
Hep.sulph	6x
Rhus.tox	6x

SCURVY
Ars.alb	30
Carb.veg	30
Merc.sol	30

SEA SICKNESS, *Travel-sickness*
Cocculus	30
Nux.vom	30
Petroleum	30

SEBACEOUS CYST
Baryt.carb	6x
Kali.iod	6x
Conium	6x

SEBORRHOEA *(dandruff) See scalp also*
Ars.alb	6x
Vinca minor	6x
Nat.mur	6x

SEMINAL VESICULITIS
Acute

Belladona	30
Merc.sol	30
Pulsatilla	30

Chronic

Agnus.castus	30
Cann.sat	30
Selenium	30

SENILE DECAY *(aging) See Adynamia, Dementia, Complaints*

Brayt.carb	6x
Conium	6x
Lycopod	6x
(Arg.nit as icr)	

SENSATIONS

Of Burning

Ars.alb	6x
Capsicum	6x
Phosphorus	6x

Of Constriction

Anacard	6x
Cactus	6x
Sulphur	6x

Of Numbness

Rhus.tox	6x
Ranun.b	6x
Kali.c	6x

SEPTICEMIA *(Also see Pyemia)*

Ars.alb	30
Baptisia	30
Chin.sul	30
(Pyrogen-200 as icr)	

SEPTICEMIA, *puerperal*

Baptisia	30
Chin.sulph	30
Rhus.tox	30
(Pyrog. as icr)	

SEPTUM, *ulceration of (nose)*

Hydrastis	30

Kali.bich	30
Silicea	30

SINUSES *(Antrum, Sphenoid, Frontal)*
General disorders
Hep.sulph	6x
Asafoetida	6x
Sticta	6x

Frontal sinuses, inflammation
Kali.bich	6x
Nux.vom	6x
Sabadilla	6x

Antrum, pain and swelling
Spigelia	6x
Phosphorus	6x
Belladona	6x

SKIN DISEASES
See Acne, Baker's itch, Barber's itch, Comedo, Ecchymoses, Frackles, Furuncles, Fungal infection, Leucoderma, Petechiae, Pityriasis, Pruritus, Psoriasis, Ringworm, Scalp, Warts.

SLEEPLESSNESS *(Insomnia)*
Coff.c	30
Gelsemium	30
Belladona	30

Due to alcohol, drugs
Gelsemium	30
Cimicifuga	30
Nux.vom	30

With arterial pulsations
Glonoine	30
Cactus	30
Belladona	30

SMALLPOX *(Variola)*
1.	Antim.tart		30
	Rhus.tox		30
	Baptisia		30
	(Merc.sol as icr)		
2.	Hep.sulph		30

Bryonia	30
Antim.tart	30
(Variolin. as icr)	

SMELL DISORDERS
Sense diminished

Cyclamen	6x
Hep.sulph	6x
Alumina	6x

Hypersensitive to flowers, food, etc

Ars.alb	6x
Colchicum	6x
Chamomilla	6x

Lost (anosmia) or perverted

Alumina	6x
Kali.bich	6x
Pulsatilla	6x

SNEEZING

1.	Ars.alb	30
	Ipecac	30
	Cepa	30
2.	Euphrasia	6x
	Gelsemium	6x
	Nux.vom	6x
3.	Sabadilla	6x
	Sticta	6x

SPERMATIC CORDS, AFFECTIONS
Pain, swelling, tenderness

1.	Arg.nit	6x
	Clematis	6x
2.	Nit.acid	6x
	Belladona	6x

SPERMATORRHOEA, *AND AFTER-EFFECTS*

1.	Cantharis	6x
	Gelsemium	6x
	Staphysagria	6x
2.	Phos.ac	6x
	Aven.sat	6x
	Anacard	6x

With debility, weak legs, backache
    China   6x
    Phos.ac   6x
    Staphysagria   6x

With emissions, premature
    Graphite   6x
    Lycopod   6x
    Caladium   6x

With erections deficient
    Calc.carb   30
    Conium   30
    Lycopod   30
(also see Impotence)

SPINAL CORD

Concussion(injury)
    Arnica   30
    Hypericum   30
    Conium   30

Hyperaesthesia
    Chin.ars   30
    Hep.sulph   30
    Ignatia   30

Hyperaesthesia, from using arms in sewing, typewriting, etc
    Cimicifuga   30
    Agaricus.m   30
    Ranun.b   30

Hyperaesthesia, sits sideways to prevent pressure on spine
    Theridion   30
    Chin.sulph   30
    Zinc.met   30

SPLEEN AFFECTIONS

Atrophy, induration
    Iodum   6x
    Agnus.castus   6x
    Phosphorus   6x

Enlargement

		Calc.ars	6x
		Ceanothus	6x
		Chin.sulph	6x

Pain

	Ceanothus	6x
	Dioscorea	6x
	Nat.mur	6x

SPRAINS, STRAINS

1.	Calc.carb	30
	Rhus.tox	30
	Ruta	30
2.	Arnica	30
	Bellis.p	30
	Hypericum	30

STAGE FRIGHT

	Gelsemium	30
	Arg.nit	30
	Anacard	30

STERILITY *(difficult or no conception)*

1.	Agnus.castus	6x
	Borax	6x
	Graphite	6x
2.	Graphite	6x
	Mur.acid	6x
	Conium	6x
	Platina	6x
3.	Nat.mur	6x
	Nat.phos	6x
	Sabal.s	6x

(Tub., Syphil., Medorr., Iod.as icr)

STOMACH, DISEASES

Dilatation (gastroptosis)

	Hydrastis	6x
	Nux.vom	6x
	Kali.bich	6x

Cardiac orifice, contraction

	Anacard	6x
	Baryt.mur	6x
	Alumina	6x

Haemorrhage (Haemetemesis)
1.	Hamamelis	30
	Millefolium	30
	Trillium	30
2.	Phosphorus	30
	Ars.alb	30
	China	30
3.	Ipecac	30
	Kreosotum	30

Pain   *See Gastric Pain*

STOMATITIS *(inflammation of mouth)*
Merc.sol	30
Borax	30
Nit.acid	30

STRABISMUS *(Squint)*
Cicuta	60
Gelsemium	60
Cyclamen	60

Convergent (eyeballs turned inwards)
Cyclamen	6x
Jaborandi	6x

Divergent (eyeballs turned outwards)
Nat.salic	6x
Morphine	6x
Cyclamen	6x

Due to worms, intestinal,
1.	Cina	6x
	Spigelia	6x
2.	Cyclamen	6x
	Santonin	6x

STRANGURY *(inflammation of urethra, prostate. bladder)*
Ars.alb	6x
Cann.sat	6x
Merc.cor	6x
Eup.purp	6x

In children

Borax	6x
Lycopod	6x
Sarsaparilla	6x

In females

Sabina	6x
Copaiva	6x
Eup.purp	6x

SUPPURATION   *See Abscess*

SURGICAL SHOCK, *anaesthetics*

Acet.acid	30
Hypericum	30

SWEAT DISORDERS

Cold, clammy

Ars.alb	6x
Carb.veg	6x
Cupr.met	6x
(Verat.alb.as icr)	

Increased.all over body

Calc.carb	6x
Pulsatilla	6x
Silicea	6x
(Merc.sol as icr)	

Increased, in axillae

Calc.carb	30
Nit.ac	30
Silicea	30

On face, forehead

Calc.carb	30
Lobel.infl	30
Varat.alb	30

On feet

Silicea	6x
Graphite	6x
Petroleum	6x

Scanty (anidrosis)

Nux.moschata	6x
Apis	6x

Convalaria	6x

SWEAT, ODOR
Foetid, offensive

Hep.sulph	6x
Merc.sol	6x
Silicea	6x

Sour, acrid

Calc.carb	6x
Hep.sulph	6x
Rheum	6x

Scanty

Nux.mos	6x
Apis	6x
Convalaria	6x

SWEAT, *affords relief, to symptoms*

Caladium	6x
Nat.mur	6x
Ars.alb	6x

SYCOSIS *See Barber's itch*

SYNCOPE *(fainting)*

Ars.alb	30
China	30
Ignatia	30
(Gelsemium as icr)	

SYNOVITIS
Acute

Rhus.tox	6x
Hep.sulph	6x
Bryonia	6x

Chronic

Rhus.tox	30
Berb.vulg	30
Merc.sol	30

SYPHILIS

Merc.sol	30
Nit.ac	30
Thuja	30
(Syphil.as icr)	

Adenopathy
  Hep.sulph 30
  Merc.sol 30
  Badiaga 30

Alopecia (hair falling)
  Ars.alb 6x
  Hep.sulph 6x
  Lycopod 6x
  (Phos. as icr)

Bone and cartilage lesions
  Asafoetida 30
  Kali.iod 30
  Mercurius 30

Condylomata
  Cinnabaris 30
  Staphysagira 30
  Thuja 30

Gummata, nodes
  Aur.met 30
  Calc.fluor 30
  Phytolacca 30

Headache
  Kali.iod 30
  Merc.sol 30
  Sarsaparilla 30

Mucous patches
  Cinnabaris 30
  Merc.sol 30
  Thuja 30

Nervous lesions
  Anacard 30
  Kali.iod 30
  Lycopod 30

Nocturnal pains
  Merc.sol 30
  Kali.iod 30
  Phytolacca 30

Rheumatism

Guaiacum	30
Merc.sol	30
Phytolacca	30

T

TABES DORSALIS *(Locomotor ataxia)*
  Alumina 6x
  Conium 6x
  Mag.phos 6x
With enuresis and urinary symptoms
  Berb.vulg 30
  Equisatum 30
  Ferr.phos 30

TACHYCARDIA *(rapid pulse)*   See Pulse
TAENIA *(tapeworm)*   See Worms
TASTE, DISORDERS
Lost
  Nat.mur 6x
  Pulsatilla 6x
  Lycopod 6x

Perverted, altered
  Merc.sol 6x
  Nux.vom 6x
  Pulsatilla 6x
  (Lycopod as icr)

Bitter, bilious
  Bryonia 6x
  Card.mar 6x
  Chelidonium 6x

Disgusting, foul
  Arnica 6x
  Carb.veg 6x
  Merc.sol 6x
  (Pulsatilla as icr)

Greasy, fatty
  Carb.veg 30
  Pulsatilla 30
  Causticum 30

TENESMUS   *Also see Strangury*

Urinary bladder
    Merc.cor   6x
    Cantharis   6x
    Lil.tig   6x

Urging painful
    Cantharis   6x
    Merc.cor   6x
    Nux.vom   6x

TEETH, AFFECTIONS

Alveolar abscess
    Hep.sul   30
    Merc.sol   30
    Carb.veg   30

Caries, decay, premature
    Calc.phos   6x
    Kreosotum   6x
    Staphysagria   6x

Caries at crown
    Mercurius   6x
    Staphysagria   6x

Craiest at root
    Mercurius   6x
    Thuja   6x
    Silicea   6x
    (Syphil. as icr)

Dentition, teething, delayed with diarrhoea
    Calc.phos   6x
    Chamomila   6x
    Podophyllum   6x

TEETH, SENSATIONS

Feel loose
    Merc.cor   6x
    Nit.acid   6x
    Carb.veg   6x

Sensitive to cold, chewing, touch
    Coff.c   30
    Staphysagria   30
    Mercurius   30

Teeth-Grinding

Cicuta	30
Podophyllum	30
Santonin	30

Toothache

Plantago	6x
Merc.sol	6x
Coff.c	6x
Staphysagria	6x

Toothache, after extraction of teeth

Arnica	30
Staphysagria	30

Pregnancy, during

Calc.carb	6x
Sepia	6x

Tobacco smoking

Selenium	6x
Spigelia	6x
Ignatia	6x

Throbbing

Merc.sol	30
Belladona	30
Glonoine	30
Silicea	30

With swelling about jaw, cheeks

Hekla.l	30
Mercurius	30
Silicea	30
(see gumboil)	

Teeth, sordes and deposits

Ailanthus	6x
Mur.ac	6x
Rhus.tox	6x
(Tub. as icr)	

TESTES, AFFECTIONS

Abscess

Hep.sulph	30
Merc.sol	30

Atrophy

Arg.nit	30

	Sabal.s	30
	Iodum	30
	(Aur.m.as icr)	

Hypertrophy
Berb.vulg	6x
Hamamelis	6x
Iodum	6x
Merc.sol	6x

Epididymitis
Belladona	6x
Clematis	6x
Mercurius	6x

Orchitis
Merc.sol	6x
Hamamelis	6x
Pulsatilla	6x

Pain
Arg.nit	6x
Belladona	6x
Conium	6x
Pulsatilla	6x

Tumor (Sarcocele)
Calc.carb	30-200
Rhodendron	30-200
Spongia	30-200

Undescended in boys
Thyroidinum	30

TETANUS *(curative and preventive)*
1.	Hypericum	30-200
	Ledum	30-200
	Nux.vom	30-200
2.	Cicuta	30-200
	Gelsemium	30-200
	Stramonium	30-200

THIRST
Excessive
Ars.alb	6x
Bryonia	6x

	Merc.cor	6x

Thirstlessness
	Apis	6x
	Gelsemium	6x
	Pulsatilla	6x

THYROID GLAND *See Goitre*

TINNITUS AURIUM *(noises in ear)*

1.		Baryt.carb	6x
		Chin.sulph	6x
2.		Kali.phos	6x
		Nat.salic	6x

Humming
Lycopod	6x
Can.sat	6x
Kali.mur	6x

Re-echoing of voice, sounds
Causticum	6x
Baryt.mur	6x
Lycopod	6x

Ringing of bells
Chin.sulph	6x
Nat.salic	6x
Graphite	6x

Whizzing
Hep.sulph	6x
Baryt.mur	6x
Belladona	6x

TOBACCO-ABUSE, *Ill-effects and to quit the habit*

Ars.alb	30
Nux.vom	30
Caladium	30

TONGUE, *Coating, Color*

Bluish
Ars.alb	6x
Secal.cor	6x
Digitalis	6x

Brownish

Ars.alb	6x
Bryonia	6x
Nat.sulph	6x

Mapped

Ars.alb	6x
Nat.mur	6x
Kali.bich	6x

Red, raw

Arum.tri	6x
Cantharis	6x
Ars.alb	6x

White, furred

Antim.c	6x
Baptisia	6x
Merc.sol	6x

Yellow, dirty, thick coating

Chelidonium	30
Merc.sol	30
Baptisia	30

TONGUE, CONDITIONS

Biting

Ignatia	6x
Phos.ac	6x

Dryness

Ars.alb	30
Bryonia	30
Nux.mos	30

TONGUE, ERUPTIONS, GROWTHS

Cancer

Ars.alb	30-200
Mur.acid	30-200
Thuja	30-200

Cracks, excoriations

Kali.bich	30
Ars.alb	30
Rhus.tox	30

Growths, nodules
    Aur.met   30
    Gall.ap   30
    Thuja   30

Ulcerations
    Merc.sol   30
    Nit.acid   30
    Arg.nit   30
    (Syphil; as icr)

TONGUE

Inflammation (Glossitis)
    Merc.sol   30
    Ars.alb   30
    Mur.acid   30

Paralysis
    Causticum   30
    Gelsemium   30
    Plumbum   30

Protrusion, difficult
    Causticum   30
    Gelsemium   30
    Ars.alb   30

Soreness
    Arum.tri   30
    Nit.acid   30
    Rhus.tox   30

TONSILS

Hypertrophy, induration
    Baryt.carb   6x
    Hep.sulph   6x
    Merc.cor   6x

Inflammation (Tonsillitis)
Acute, follicular
    Baryt.carb   6x
    Merc.sol   6x
    Phytolacca   6x

Acute (Quinsy)
    Baryt.carb   6x
    Hep.sulph   6x
    Merc.sol   6x

TRACHOMA   *See Eyes, Granular lids*

TRICHOPHYTOSIS   *See Ringworm*

TRISMUS *(lockjaw, stiffness)*
    Cicuta   30-200
    Hypericum   30-200
    Nux.vom   30-200

TUBERCULOSIS
    Ars.iod   30
    China   30
    Ipecac   30

Diarrhoea
    Ars.alb   30
    China   30
    Phosphorus   30

Digestive disorders
    Cupr.ars   30
    Hydrastis   30
    Nux.vom   30

Dyspnoea
    Ipecac   30
    Carb.veg   30
    Phosphorus   30

Emaciation
    Ars.alb   30
    Iodum   30
    Calc.phos   30

Fever
    Baptisia   30
    Chin.ars   30
    Ferr.phos   30

Haemoptysis
1.   Acal.ind   30-200

	Ferr.phos	30-200
2.	Hamamelis	30-200
	Ipecac	30-200

TUMORS
Cystic
Baryt.carb	30
Kali.brom	30
Iodum	30

Bone like protuberances
Hekla.l	30
Calc.fluor	30
Lapis.alb	30

Fibroid, bleeding
Hydras.mur	30
Trillium	30
Sabina	30

Lipoma
Baryt.carb	6x
Lapis.alb	6x
Thuja	6x

Ploypi
Phosphorus	30
Silicea	30
Kali.sulph	30

TYPHOID FEVER
1.	Baptisia	30
	Gelsemium	30
	Rhus.tox	30
2.	Bryonia	30
	Carb.veg	30
	Lycopod	30
	(Pyrogen.as icr)	

TYPHOID FEVER, CONCOMITANTS
Delerium
Belladona	30
Hyoscyamus	30
Stramonium	30

Diarrhoea
    Ars.alb   30
    Cupr.met   30
    Merc.sol   30

Ecchymoses
    Arnica   30
    Ars.alb   30
    Carb.veg   30

Epistaxis
    Hamamelis   30
    Ipecac   30
    Bryonia   30

Headache
1.   Belladona   30
    Bryonia   30
2.   Gelsemium   30
    Nux.vom   30

Haemorrhage
1.   Baptisia   30
    Hamamelis   30
2.   Millefolium   30
    Nit.acid   30

Pneumonia, bronchial symptoms
    Antim.tart   30
    Bryonia   30
    Ipecac   30
    (Sulphur.as icr)

U

ULCER

Bleeding, easily, when touched
Carb.veg	30
Nit.acid	30
Phosphorus	30

Deep
Asafoetida	30
Nit.acid	30
Kali.bich	30

Eroding, of face — Conium

Fistulous
Calc.fluor	30
Nit.acid	30
Silicea	30

Scrofulous
Calc.carb	30
Hep.sulph	30
Silicea	30
(Sulphur.as icr)	

Sensitive
Arnica	30
Hep.sulph	30
Nit.acid	30

Traumatic
Arnica	30
Conium	30
(externally, Calendula Q)	

Varicose
Hamamelis	30
Carb.veg	30
Fl. acid	30

ULCER *with base, blue or black*
Ars.alb	30
Calc.fluor	30
Lachesis	30

With discharge, fetid, purulent
　　　　　Carb.veg　　　　　　　　　30
　　　　　Hep.sulph　　　　　　　　30
　　　　　Merc.cor　　　　　　　　　30

　　　With, edges, deep punched out
　　　　　Kali.bich　　　　　　　　　30
　　　　　Phosphorus　　　　　　　　30
　　　With, edges, irregular
　　　　　Merc.sol　　　　　　　　　30
　　　　　Nit.acid　　　　　　　　　30

UMBILICUS
　　　Bleeding from, in newborn
　　　　　Calc.phos　　　　　　　　6x30
　　　　　Abrotanum　　　　　　　　6x30
　　　Pain, soreness
　　　　　Calc.phos　　　　　　　　　30
　　　　　Carb.veg　　　　　　　　　30
　　　　　Chamomilla　　　　　　　　30

URAEMIA
　　　　　Cupr.ars　　　　　　　　　30
　　　　　Helleborus　　　　　　　　30
　　　　　Terebenthina　　　　　　　30
　　　Coma
　　　　　Am.c　　　　　　　　　　　30
　　　　　Helleborus　　　　　　　　30
　　　　　Morphine　　　　　　　　　30
　　　Convulsions
　　　　　Cicuta　　　　　　　　　30-200
　　　　　Cupr.ars　　　　　　　　30-200
　　　　　Merc.cor　　　　　　　　30-200
　　　Vomiting
　　　　　Ars.alb　　　　　　　　　　30
　　　　　Kreosotum　　　　　　　　　30
　　　　　Nux.vom　　　　　　　　　　30

URETHRA
Burning
	Cantharis	30
	Merc.cor	30
	Cann.sat	30

Burning, between acts of urination
	Berb.vulg	30
	Cann.sat	30
	Staphysagria	30

Haemorrhage
	Lycopod	30
	Calc.carb	30

Urethritis (inflammation) See Gonorrhoea also
	Cantharis	30
	Copaiva	30
	Thuja	30

Itching
	Petrosel	30
	Arg.nit	30
	Merc.cor	30

Stricture, Organic
	Cantharis	30
	Sul.iod	30
	Clematis	30

Urethral Fever (due to catheter)
	Chin.ars	30
	Aconite	30
	Gelsemium	30

URINARY FLOW, DESIRE
Constant desire
	Cantharis	30
	Sabal.s	30
	Cann.sat	30

Frequent desire
	Chimphila	30
	Nux.vom	30
	Causticum	30

Frequent desire, at night

Causticum	30
Phose.acid	30
Sulphur	30

Irresistable, Sudden desire

Cantharis	30
Merc.cor	30
Petros	30

URINARY FLOW

Intermittent flow

Conium	30
Hep.sulph	30
Sabal.s	30

Involuntary

Arg.nit	30
Causticum	30
Gelsemium	30

Involuntary, at night

Causticum	30
Kreosotum	30
Sulphur	30

When coughing, sneezing

Causticum	30
Sulphur	30
Zinc.met	30

URINE, RETENTION OF *(Ischiuria)*

From inflammation

Aconite	30
Cantharis	30
Plusatilla	30

From paralysis

Causticum	30
Opium	30
Plumb.met	30

From delivery (after Labor)

Hyoscyamus	30
Opium	30
Arnica	30

From prostatic hypertrophy

Chimaphila	30

Digitalis	30
Zinc.met	30

From surgical operations

Causticum	30
Aconite	30
Nux.vom	30

URINE, SCANTY FLOW

Berb.vulg	30
Chimaphila	30
Juniperus	30

Drop by drop

Cantharis	30
Merc.cor	30
Sabal.s	30

URINE, SUPPRESSION *(Anuria)*

Apis	30
Cantharis	30
Helleborus	30

URINATION

Complaints before act

Cantharis	30
Berb.vulg	30
Lyccopod	30

Complaints during act

Merc.cor	30
Arg.nit	30
Equisatum	30

Complaints after act

Capsicum	30
Kreosotum	30
Thuja	30

URINE, *Sensation as if urine remained behind*

Berb.vulg	30
Hep.sulph	30
Kali.bich	30

Tenesmus, urging, straining

Cantharis	30

	Equisatum	30
	Staphysagria	30

URINE, TYPES
Acid
	Benz.acid	30
	Merc.cor	30
	Sarsaparilla	30

Alkaline
	Kali.acet	30
	Phos.acid	30
	Mag.phos	30

Albuminuric See Abuminuria

Bloody, hemoglobinuria
	Berb.vulg	30
	Hamamelis	30
	Millefolium	30

Burning, hot
	Borax	30
	Cantharis	30
	Merc.cor	30

Oily, Pellicle
	Cort.t	30
	Iodum	30
	Phosphorus	30

Milky
	Phos.acid	30
	Cina	30
	Viola.od	30

Red, dark
	Aconite	30
	Bryonia	30
	Kali.bich	30

URINE, ODOR
Pungent, ammoniacal
	Borax	30
	Nit.acid	30
	Pareira.b	30

Sharp, strong
	Benz.acid	30

	Chin.sulph	30
	Lycopod	30
Sour		
	Graphite	30
	Petroleum	30
	Solidago	30

URINE, SEDIMENT-TYPES

Bile
- Chelidonium — 30
- Chionanthus — 30
- Nat.sulph — 30

Casts
- Ars.alb — 30
- Cantharis — 30
- Plumbum — 30

Cells, debris
- Berb.vulg — 30
- Cantharis — 30
- Merc.cor — 30

Chlorides, diminished
- Baryt.mur — 30
- Chelidonium — 30
- Copaiva — 30

Grayish white, granular
- Graphite — 30
- Berb.vulg — 30
- Cantharis — 30

Oxalates
- Berb.vulg — 30
- Kali.sulph — 30
- Nat.phos — 30

Pus
- Cantharis — 30
- Hep.sulph — 30
- Merc.cor — 30

URTICARIA *(Hives)*
- Urtica u — 30

Nat.mur	30
Sulphur	30

From emotions

Anacard	30
Ignatia	30
Kali.brom	30

From gastric derangements

Plusatilla	30
Antim.c	30
Ars.alb	30

From menstrual conditions

Cimicifuga	30
Plusatilla	30
Dulcamara	30

Seuqellae, from suppressed hives

Apis	30
Urt.u	30

UTERUS

Atony, weakness

Alet.f	30
Caulophyllum	30
Sepia	30

Cervix, inflammation

Merc.cor	30
Ars.alb	30
Sepia	30
Belladona	30

Cervix, tumors

Kreosotum	30
Thuja	30
Carb.an	30
Iodum	30

Fibroids

Aur.iod	30
Calc.carb	30
Conium	30

Displacements, prolapsus

Alet.f	30

Aur.m. n	30
Calc.carb	30

Inflammation (Metritis)

Merc.cor	30
Ars.alb	30
Sepia	30

Pain, bruised broken feeling

Aesculus	30
Trillium	30
Arnica	30

Pain, pressing, as if viscera would protrude out

Sepia	30
Kreosotum	30
Lil.tig	30

V

VACCINATION, *injection, ill-effects*
	Thuja	30
	Silicea	30
	Merc.sol	30

VAGINA, AFFECTIONS OF
Aphthous, erosions
	Arg.nit	30
	Helonias	30
	Sepia	30

Inflammation (Vaginitis)
Acute
	Cantharis	30
	Kreosotum	30
	Merc.cor	30

Chronic
	Calc.carb	30
	Sepia	30
	Kreosotum	30

Prolapse
	Lappa	30
	Sepia	30
	Belladona	30

VULVA-LABIA
Abscess (Vulvo-vaginitis)
	Hep.sulph	30
	Merc.cor	30
	Silicea	30

Itching
	Ambra.grisea	30
	Caladium	30
	Sulphur	30

VALVULAR DISEASES, OF HEART
1.	Cactus	1x-6x
	Cratagus	1x-6x

2. Digitalis — 1x-6x
Glonoine — 30

VARICOCELE
Ferr.phos — 30
Hamamelis — 30
Pulsatilla — 30

VARICOSE ULCERS *(See Ulcer)*

VEINS, AFFECTIONS OF
Engorged, distended
Hamamelis — 30
Carb.veg — 30
Aloes — 30

Inflamed (Phlebitis)
Hamamelis — 30
Pulsatilla — 30
Ars.alb — 30

Inflamed, chronic
Merc.cor — 30
Pulsatilla — 30
Arnica — 30

Varicosed
Calc.carb — 6x
Card.m — 6x
Hamamelis — 6x
Carb.veg — 6x

VERTIGO, TYPES
Anaemia of brain (ischemia)
Conium — 30
Cocculus — 30
China — 30

Gastro-enteric derangements
Bryonia — 6x
Cocculus — 6x
Nux.vom — 6x
Pulsatilla — 6x

Old age (senile)
Ambra.grisea — 30

Conium	30
Phosphorus	30

When riding in car

Cocculus	30
Hep.sulph	30
Petroleum	30

When walking

Causticum	30
Gelsemium	30
Belladona	30

VISION, DISORDERS

AMAUROSIS (Blindness)

Gelsemium	30
Merc.cor	30
Phosphorus	30

BLINDNESS, sudden, due to retrobulbar neuritis, optic neuritis   See Neuritis

COLOR-BLINDNESS

Benz.dinit	30
Santonin	30
Physostigma	30

DAY-BLINDNESS

Bothrops	30
Lycopod	30
Phosphorus	30

NIGHT-BLINDNESS

Belladona	30
Nux.vom	30
Physostigma	30

AMBLYOPIA (Blurred, weak vision)

Ruta	30
Gelsemium	30
Nat.mur	30

DIPLOPIA (double vision)

Belladona	30
Cyclamen	30
Gelsemium	30

HEMIOPIA (one half visible)

Lith.carb	30
Titanium	30
Calc.sulph	30

SHORT-SIGHTEDNESS (weak distant vision)
                              See Myopia

FAR-SIGHTEDNESS (weak near vision)
                              See Hypermetropia

VITREOUS OPACITIES

Hamamelis	30
Merc.cor	30
Thuja	30

VOMITING

Drinks of any kind

Ars.alb	30
Cantharis	30
Ipecac	30

Eating, drinking

Ipecac	30
Ars.alb	30
Bryonia	30

Gastric irritation

Ars.alb	30
Nux.vom	30
Ipecac	30
Pulsatilla	30

Milk

Aethusa	30
Mag.carb	30
Merc.sol	30

Pregnancy

Ipecac	30
Sepia	30

VOMITING, TYPE

Acid, sour

Calc.carb	30
Iris.v	30
Nat.phos	30

Bilious (green, yellow)

Bryonia	30

Card.mar	30
Chelidomium	30

Bloody

Ars.alb	30
Ferr.phos	30
Hamamelis	30

With collapse, weakness

Ars.alb	30
Tabacum	30
Lobel.infl	30

With fruitless retching

Bismuth	30
Ars.alb	30
Cupr.m	30

W

WARMTH, *ameliorates See Amelioration*
WARTS *(Verruca)*
   Bleed easily, large
Nit.acid	30
Cinnabaris	30
Causticum	30

   Condylomata, fig-warts
Thuja	30
Nit.acid	30
Lycopod	30

   Situated on body, anywhere
Nat.sulph	30
Sepia	30

   On face, hands
Causticum	30
Dulcamara	30
Kali.c	30

   On genito-anal surface
Nit.acid	30
Thuja	30

WEAKNESS, SHOCK *See Adynamia*
WHOOPING COUGH *See Pertussis*
WORM FEVER
Cina	30
Merc.cor	30
Santonin	30

WORMS, *intestinal*
   Ascaris lumbricoides
Cina	30
Santonin	30
Teucrium	30

   Oxyuris vermicularis
Cina	30
Merc.sol	30
Santonin	30

Taenia
    Filix.m 30
    Granatum 30
    Merc.sol 30

WOUNDS

Bleed profusely
    Hamamelis 30
    Millefolium 30
    Arnica 30
    (Crot.t-200 as icr)

Bullet, from
    Arnica 30
    Calendula 30

Incised; surgical operation
    Arnica 30
    Hypericum 30
    Staphysagria 30

With gangrenous tendency
    Calendula 30
    Sulphur 30
    Ars.alb 30

(Calendula.Q for external and internal use)

WRIST AFFECTIONS

Ganglion on back
    Benz.acid 30
    Ruta 30
    Silicea 30

Pains
    Act.spicata 30
    Cauloph 30
    Ruta 30

Cramps, painful spasm (Writer's cramps)
    Causticum 30
    Cupr.met 30
    Ruta 30

Rheumatic
    Causticum 30

	Ruta	30
	Sabina	30
Paralysis		
	Plumb.met	30
	Conium	30
	Ruta	30

Abbreviations Table

A	
Abies.n	Abies nigra
Acon.lyco	Aconite lycoton
Acon. n	Aconitum napellus
Aethusa	Aehtusa cynapium
Agaricus. m	Agaricus muscarius
Agnus. c	Agnus castus
Agraph.n	Agraphis nutans
Alet. f	Aletris farinosa
Allium. c	Allium cepa
Allium. s	Allium sativam
Am. carb	Ammonium carb
Amyg. pers	Amygdalus persica
Amyl. nit	Amyl nitrite
Anacard	Anacardium
Anthracin	Anthracinum
Antim. c	Antimonium crudum
Antim. tart	Antimonium tartaricum
Apis	Apis mellifica
Apocy. c	Apocynum cannabinum
Aran. d	Aranea diadema
Arg. m	Argentum metallicum
Arg.nit	Argentum nitricum
Ars. alb	Arsenicum album
Ars. brom	Arsenicum bromatum
Ars.sul.fl	Ars sulph. flavum
Arum. tri	Arum triphyllum
Asarum	Asarum Europium
Asterias. rub	Asterias rubins
Aur. iod	Aurum iodatum
Aur. met	Aurum metallicum
Aur. mur	Aurum muriaticum
Aur. m. n	Aurum mur. natronatum
Avena. s	Avena sativa

B	
Bacil	Bacillinum
Baryt. carb	Baryta carb
Baryt. mur	Baryta muriaticum
Bell	Belladona
Bellis. p	Bellis perennis
Benz. ac	Benzonic acid
Benz. dinit	Benzin dinitric
Berb. aquifol	Berberis aquifolium
Berb. vulg	Berberis vulgaris
Bismuth	Bismuthum
Bothrops. l	Bothrops lanciolatus
Bry	Bryonia
C	
Cadm. sul	Cadmium sulph
Calc. ars	Calcarea arsenica
Calc. carb	Calcarea carbonica
Calc. fluor	Calcarea fluorica
Calc. phos	Calcarea phosphorica
Calc. pic	Calcarea picrata
Calc. renalis	Calcarea renalis
Cann. ind	Cannabis indica
Cann. sat	Cannabis sativa
Canth	Cantharis
Carbol. ac	Carbolic acid
Carb. an	Carbo animalis
Carbo.veg	Carbo vegetablis
Carcinocin	Carcinocin
Card. m	Carduus marianus
Cauloph	Caulophyllum
Ceanothus	Ceanothus Americana
Cepa	Allium cepa
Chimaphila. u	Chimaphila umbelata
China	Cinchina officinalis
Chin. ars	China arsenicosum
Chin. sulph	China sulphuricum
Cicuta	Cicuta virosa

Cinchona	Cinchona officinalis
Clematis	Clematis erecta
Coff. c	Coffea cruda
Colocynth	Colocynthis
Crot. h	Crotalus horridus
Crot. tig	Croton tiglium
Cupr. acet	Cuprum aceticum
Cupr. ars	Cuprum arsenicum
Cupr. met	Cuprum metallicum

D

Diosc	Dioscorea
Dros	Drosera

E

Elaps	Elaps corallinus
Epigea	Epigea repens
Eupat. prf	Eupatorium perfoliatum
Eup. purp	Eupatorium purpurim

F

Ferr. phos	Ferrum phosphoricum
Ferr. pic	Ferrum picricum
Fluor. ac	Fluoric acid
Fucus. v	Fucus vesiculosis

G

Galium. ap	Galium aparine
Gels	Gelsemium
Glon	Glonoine

H

Hekla. l	Hekla lava
Helleb	Helleborus niger
Hep. sulph	Hepar sulphuris
Hippoz	Hippozaeninum
Hoang. n	Hoang nan
Hydrocy. ac	Hydrocyanic acid

I

icr	Inter-current remedy
Iris.v	Iris versicolor
J	
Jaborandi	Pilocarpus microphyllus
Jugl. c	Juglans cinerea
Juniperus	Juniperus communis
K	
Kali. ars	Kali arsenicum
Kali. bich	Kali bichromicum
Kali. brom	Kali bromatum
Kali. c	Kali carbonicum
Kali. cyan	Kali cyanatum
Kali. iod	Kali hydroiodicum
Kali. mur	Kali muriaticum
Kali. permang	Kali permanganum
Kali. phos	Kali phosphoricum
L	
Lac.can	Lac caninum
Lach	Lachesis
Lapis. alb	Lapis albus
Lathyr	Lathyrus
Lauroc	Laurocerasus
Lemna. m	Lemna minor
Lil. tig	Lilium tigrinum
Lith. carb	Lithium carbonicum
Lobel. infl	Lobelia inflata
Lycopod	Lycopodium
M	
Mag. carb	Magnesia carbonica
Mag. mur	Magnesia muriatica
Mag. phos	Magnesia phosphorica
Mang	Manganum
Mang. ox	Manganum ox
Medorr	Medorrhinum
Merc. cor	Mercurialis corrosive
Merc.cyn	Merc. cyanatus

Merc. dulcis	Merc. dulcis
Merc. i. r	Merc. iodatus rub
Merc. v	Merc. vivus
Merc. sol	Merc. solubilis
Mezer	Mezereum
Mur. ac	Muriatic acid
Myristca. s	Myristica sebifera

N

Naja	Naja tripudians
Nat.c	Natrum carbonicum
Nat. mur	Natrum muriaticum
Nat. phos	Natrum phosphoricum
Nat. sulph	Natrum sulphuricum
Nit. acid	Nitric acid
Nux. mos	Nux moschata
Nux. vom	Nux. vomica

O

Ocim. can	Ocimum canum
Oenanthe	Oenanthe crocata
Oophor	Oophorinum
Op	Opium
Orchitin	Orchitinum

P

Petros	Petroselinum
Phos. ac	Phosphoric acid
Pic. ac	Picric acid
Plumb. iod	Plumbum iodatum
Pop.tr	Populus tremuloides
Prim. ob	Primula obconia
Prun. s	Prunus spinosa
Psorin	Psorinum
Puls	Pulsatilla nigricans
Pyrogen	Pyrogenium

R

Ranun. b	Ranunculus bulbosus
Rhus. tox	Rhus toxicodendron

S

Sabad	Sabadilla
Sabal. s	Sabal serrulata
Sambucus	Sambucus nigra
Sarsap	Sarsaparilla
Scirrhin	Scirrhinum
Secal. cor	Secale cornutum
Selen	Selenium
Sil	Silicea
Spongia	Spongia tosta
Stramon	Stramonium
Stront. c	Strontia carb
Strych. n	Strych. nitricum
Sul	Sulphur
Sul. ac	Sulphuric acid
Sul. iod	Sulphur iodatum
Syphil	Syphilinum

T

Tab	Tabacum
Tarax	Taraxicum
Tellur	Tellurium
Tereb	Terebinthina
Thlaspi	Thlaspi bursa pastoris
Tub	Tuberculinum

U

Uran. Nit	Uranium nitricum
Uric. ac	Uric acid
Urtica. u	Urtica urens

V

Variolin	Variolinum
Verat. alb	Veratrum album
Verat. v	Veratrum viride
Vespa.c	Vespa crabro

Vib.op	Viburnum opulus
Z	
Zinc. cy	Zincum cyanatum
Zinc. met	Zincum metallicum

A

	Page
Abdomen	1
Abortion	1,2
Abscess	2

Acid, pickles, excessive desire See appetite perverted
Acidity, gastric.... Also see Pyrosis and Dyspepsia 2

Acne	2
Actinomycosis	3
Addison's disease	3
Adenitis (lymph node inflammation)	3,4
Adenoids	See Adenitis
Adenopathy, syphilitic	See Syphilis
Adynamia, collapse, weakness	4
Aggravations – causations	5
Aging, effects of	See Senile Deacy, Dementia, Adynamia
Air, cool, must have windows open	See Ameliorations
Air, cool, dry, aggravates	See Aggravations
Air, cool, open, ameliorates	See Ameliorations
Albuminuria	See kidney
Albuminuria, during pregnancy	See Pregnancy
Alcoholism	See Delirium
Alopecia	See Scalp, Ringworm
Alopecia, syphilitic	See Syphilis
Ameliorations	9
Amenorrhoea	See Menstruation
Anaemia	11
Anasarca (generalised oedema of body)	See Oedema
Angina pectoris	See Heart diseases
Anidrosis (absence of sweating)	See Sweat disorders
Anthropophobia (fear of human beings)	See Fears
Anuria (suppression of urinary output)	See Urine

Anxiety	See Moods
Apathetic, indifferent to everything	See Moods
Appetite-perverted cravings (Pica), excessive desires	13
Appetite-aversions (things that disagree)	12
Aphthae (white painful oral ulcers)	See Mouth, inflammation
Arthritis	See Rheumatism
Ascaris	See Worms
Ascites	See Oedema
Asphyxia	14
Asthenopia (weakness of eyes)	See Eyes, Amblyopia, Myopia, Hypermetropia
Asthma	See Dyspnoea
Atony, urinary bladder	See Bladder
Aversions	See Appetite-things that disagree
Aversion to physical and mental work, indecisive	See Moods
Axilla	14

B

Backache	15
Back, Weakness	16
Baker's itch (Lichen)	16
Barber's itch	16
Basedow's Disease	16
Bed sores (decubitus)	16,17
Bell's palsy or paralysis	17
Bending double, ameliorates	See Ameliorations
Bending forward aggravates	See Aggravations
Biliary colic	17
Biliousness	17
Bladder, urinary	17,18,19
Blepharitis	See Eyelids 19
Blindness (amaurosis)	See Vision

Blisters		20
Blood deficiency	See Anaemia	20
Blood disorders		19
Blood purifier, formula		20
Blood and lymphatic disorders		20
Blood pressure	See Hypertension	
Body, as a whole		20
Bone affections		21
Bones and cartilages, lesions	See Syphilis	
Bowel obstruction, intussusception		22
Brachialgia (neuralgia)	See Neuralgia	
Brain, diseases of		22,23
Brain – fag		23
Breasts	See Mammary glands, Climacteric disorders, Menstruation, Pregnancy.	
Breath, cold; offensive		23
Bright's disease	See Nephritis	
Bromidrosis (offensive sweat)	See Sweat	
Bronchiectasis		23
Bronchitis		24
Bruises	See Injuries	
Bubo		24
Bulbar paralysis		24
Bunions		24
Burns, scalds		24
Bursitis, synovitis, knee joints		24
Butter, disagrees	See Appetite	

C

Cabbage, disagrees	See Appetite	
Calculi, biliary		25
Calculi, renal	See Kidney	

Cancer	25,26
Carbuncle, anthrax	26
Cardiac asthma	See Dyspnoea, cardiac
Cardiac dropsy	See Oedema
Cardiac neuroses	26
Cardialgia (pain at cardiac orifice of stomach)	26
Cardiac orifice, contraction, reflux oesophagitis	26
Caries, bones	See Bones, Necrosis
Cartilage, peri – chondritis	26
Catalepsy, trance, hypnosis	26
Cataract	27
Catheterism (catheter-fever)	27
Cellulitis	27
Cerebro-spinal meningitis	See Meningitis
Cervical spondylosis	See Neuralgia
Chancre	27
Charocoal, chalk-excessive desire	See Appetite
Checked discharges, ill-effects from	27
Cheeks, yellow saddle	28
Cheeks, diseases of	See Face
Chicken-pox	28
Chillblains	28
Chilliness	28
Chloasma	28
Chlorosis	See Anaemia
Cholera	28
Cholera infantum-Summer complaint	28,29
Chorea (St. Vitus Dance)	29
Ciliary neuralgia	See Neuralgia
Cirrhosis of liver	See Liver, atrophy
Clairvoyance	29
Clergyman's sore throat	29
Climacteric disturbances	30
Coccyx	31

Coffee-excessive desire	See Appetite	
Coitus, aggravates	See Aggravation	
Cold, Coryza	See Rhinitis	
Colic-types		31
Colic-aggravations		32
Colic-ameliorations		33
Colic-biliary (also see calculi, biliary)		33
Colic-renal	See Kidney	
Cold-ameliorates	See Ameliorations	
Collapse	See Adynamia	
Color-blindness	See Vision disorders	
Coma		33
Comedo		33
Complaints, symptoms-types of		33
Condylomata	See Warts	
Conjunctivitis	See Eyes	
Constipation-types, concomitants		34
Convulsions	Also see Epilepsy	34
Cornea		36
Callosities, corns		36
Coryza, colds		36,37
Cough		38
Cowperitis		38
Cracked lips, ulcerations		38
Cramps		38
Cretinism		38
Cyanosis		38
Cystitis	See Bladder	
Cysts, ovarian		39
Cysts, sebaceous		39
Cystic tumors		39

D

Damp, living houses, aggravates	See Aggravations
Dandruff	See Seborrhoea

Deafness	40
Debility	See Adynamia
Decubitus	See Bed sores
Delerium (psychological diseases)	40
Delivery, easy	41
Dementia	41
Dengue fever	41
Dentition	41
Depression	41
Dermatitis	See Pruritus and Skin diseases
Diabetes insipidus	42
Diabetes mellitus	42
Diaphragm, inflammation	42
Diarrhoea-dysentery	42,43,44
Diphtheria	44
Diplopia	See Vision
Drinks, warm, ameliorate	See Ameliorations
Dropsy	See Oedema
Drowsiness, after meals	44
Drugs, diets-abuse	44,45
Duodenum, inflammation, ulcer	45
Dysentery	See Diarrhoea also 45
Dysmenorrhoea	46
Dyspepsia	46,47,48
Dysphagia	48
Dyspnoea (difficult breathing; Bronchial Asthma)	48
Dyspnoea, cardiac	50
Dysuria	50

E

Ear diseases	See Earache, External auditory canal, Otitis, Otorrhoea, Otalgia
Earache	51
Ecchymoses	51

Eclampsia		51
Eczema	See Pruritus	119
Ectropion	See Eyes	
Elephantiasis		51
Emissions, seminal		51,52
Encephalitis lethargica (sleeping sickness)		52
Endocarditis	See Heart	
Endocervicitis	See Uterus	
Endometritis	See Uterus	
Enteralgia	See Colic	
Enteritis	See Diarrhoea	
Entropion	See Eyes	
Enuresis	See Urine, Bladder	
Epididymitis	See Testicles	
Epilepsy		52
Epiphora		53
Epistaxis	See nose	
Epithelioma		53
Erratic, changing, shifting symptoms	See Aggravations	
Erotomania	See Mania	
Eructations	See Dyspepsia	
Erysipelas (acute streptococcal cellulitis of skin)		53,54
Erythema		54
Eustachean deafness	See Deafness	
Excesses, vital drains	See Aggravation	
Exophthalmic goitre	*See goitre*	
Exertion makes worse	See Aggravation	
Exercise, ameliorates	See Amelioration	
Exostoses (a benign cartilage capped swelling on bone)		
Expectoration, ameliorates	See Amelioration	
External auditory canal, diseases		54
Eyes, affections		55
Eyelids, growths, inflammation		55

F

Face, appearance	57
Face, bones	57
Face, diseases of	58
Face, sensations	59
Fainting	See Syncope
Fannned, being, ameliorates	See Amelioration
Fasting, ameliorates	See Amelioration
Fats, aggravate	See Aggravation
Fears	59
Feet, in ice water, ameliorates	See Amelioration
Felon (whitlow, panaritium)	59
Fever	60
Fibroids, tumors	*See tumors*
Fish, aggravates	See Aggravation
Fistula dentalis	See Teeth, Caries
Food of any kind, disagrees	See Appetite-aversions
Food poisoning (decayed food)	See Poisoning
Flatulence	See Dyspepsia, Indigestion
Fractures	See Bones
Frackles (lentigo)	See Face
Furuncle (boil)	61
Fungal infections	See Pityriasis, Actinomycosis, Ringworm

G

Gait disorders	62
Galactorrhoea	62
Gall-stones	See Calculi, biliary
Gall-stones, colic	See Colic, biliary
Ganglion, on back of wrist	62
Gangrene	62
Gas fumes, ill effects	63
Gastric pain	63

Gastritis (inflammation of gastric mucosa)	63
Genital warts	See Penis, warts
Gingivitis (inflammation of gums)	See Gums
Gleet (chronic gonorrhoea)	64
Glossitis (inflammation of tongue)	See Tongue
Goitre	65
Gonorrhoea (specific urethritis)	66
Gout	66
Grief, ill effects	See Aggravation
Grief, aggravates	See Aggravation
Gums	66

H

Hay fever	See Rhinitis, Sneezing
Headache	68, 69
Headache, syphilitic	See Syphilis
Head, wrapped up warm, ameliorates	See Amelioration
Heartburn	See Pyrosis
Heart diseases	70
Heat, ameliorates	See Amelioration
Hematuria (blood in urine)	See Urine 73
Hemetamesis (blood in vomiting)	73
Hemoglobinuria	See Urine
Hemophilia	73
Hemorrhage (bleeding)	74
Hemorrhoids, piles	74
Hemoptysis (blood-spitting with cough)	74
Hepatitis	See Liver, inflammation
Hoarseness, aphonia	See Coryza
Hodgkin's disease	75
Hypermetropia (far-sightedness)	75
Hypertension	75
Hyperthyroidism	See Goitre

Hypochondriacal tendency   See Neurasthenia
Hypothyroidism   See Goitre

I

Impetigo   76
Impotence (also see Penis, Emissions, Spermatorrhoea,
        Adynamia)   76
Indigestion   *See dyspepsia*
Infertility in females   See Sterility
Inflammation   76
Influenza (see Coryza, Cough, Pharyngitis, Bronchitis) 76
Ingrown toe-nail   See Nails
Inguinal lymph node (adenitis)   See Adenitis
Injuries and after-effects   76
Insanity   (see Mania, Memory, Moods, e.g., anxiety,
            apathetic, delerium)
Insect bites   77
Insomnia (sleeplessness)   See Sleeplessness
Intercostal neuralgia   See Neuralgia
Intertrigo (chaffing)   See Erythema
Intestines, obstruction, ulcer   22, 77
Iris, prolapse   78
Iritis   78
Itching, dermatitis   See Pruritus

J

Jaundice   79
Jaws   79
Joints   See Rheumatism   80

K

Kidney diseases (also see Pyelitis)	81
Kidney stones	82
Keloid	83
Keratitis (inflammation of cornea)	83

L

Lacrimation	See Epiphora	
Lactation		84
Labor, disorders		84
Labor, easy remedy		84
Laryngitis		84
Lice infestation	(also see phthriasis)	113
Leucoderma (vitiligo)		85
Lichen	See Baker's itch	
Light, aggravates	See Aggravation	
Lips	See Mouth, external	
Leukaemia		85
Leucocytosis		85
Legs		85
Legs, neuritis	See Neuritis	86
Leucorrhoea		86
Lice		88
Liver diseases		87
Lipoma (fatty tumor)		88
Localised symptoms	See Aggravation	
Locomotor ataxia	See Tabes dorsalis; Gait	88
Lumbago	See Backache	
Lungs		88
Lying down, aggravates	See Aggravation	
Lying down, ameliorates	See Amelioration	
Lying down on left side, aggravates	See Aggravation	
Lying down on left side, ameliorates	See Amelioration	
Lying down on right side, aggravates	See Aggravation	

Lying down on right side, ameliorates See Amelioration
Lying down on painful side ameliorates See Amelioration
Lymph nodes See Adenitis
Lymphatic system formula See Blood

M

Malaria	90
Mammary glands, affections	90
Mania	90
Marasmus (malnutrition)	91
Mastoid disease	91
Masturbation, ill effects	91
Measles	91
Meat, excessive desire	See Appetite
Migraine	92
Milk, aggravates	See Aggravation
Misdeeds of others	See Aggravation
Memory	92
Menopause	See Climacteric
Menstruation disorders	92,93
Mental exertion, aggravates	See Aggravation
Meniere's disease	See Vertigo 94
Meningitis	94
Metrirtis, endometritis	94
Metrorrhagia	95
Moods, phychiatric diseases	95
Morning sickness	See Pregnancy
Morphine habit, opium, Heroin addiction	95
Mortification from an offence	See Aggravation
Mouth (internal, external, lips)	96
Motion, aggravates	See Aggravation
Mucous patches	See Syphilis
Mumps (parotitis)	97
Muscae volitantes (spots before eyes)	See Optical illusions

Muscles	98
Myelitis	98
Myopia (short-sightedness)	98
Myxoedema (hypothyroidism) See Goitre also	99

N

Nails	100
Narcotics, aggravate	See Aggravation
Nasal polyp	See Polyp and nose
Nausea	101
Necrosis	101
Nephritis	See Kidneys
Nephro-lithiasis	See Kidneys
Nervous lesions, syphilitic	See Syphilis
Neuralgia	101
Neurasthenia (nervous prostration)	See Adynamia also
Neuritis	103
Night, aggravates	See Aggravation
Night-blindness	See Vision disorders
Night-terrors	103
Nipples	103
Nocturnal pains	See Syphilis
Nodosities (tophi)	103
Nose, diseases of	103, 104, 105
Nostalgia (home-sickness)	105
Nymphomania (excessive sex desire in women)	105

O

Obesity	106
Oedema (dropsy)	106
Oesophagus	106
Oesophagitis, reflux	See Cardialgia

Old age, effects, impotence	See Adynamia, Dementia, Senile decay	106
One half of body	See Aggravation	
Ophthalmia (inflammation of eyes, esp. the onjunctiva)		106
Optic nerve		107
Optical illusions		107
Osteo-myelitis		107
Otitis media (middle ear infection)		108
Otorrhoea (ear discharge)		108
Otalgia (pain in ear)		108
Ovaries		108,109
Ovarian cycts		109

P

Palate		110
Palpitation	See Heart	
Panaritium, whitlow of finger nail	See Felon, Nail Inflammation	110
Pancreas, diseases		110
Paralysis (also see Gait disorders)		110,111
Paraplegia	See Paralysis	111
Parkinsonism	See Paralysis	110
Parotitis (Mumps)		111
Pastry, disagrees	See Appetite	
Pelvic diseases		111
Pemphigus		112
Penis, diseases		112
Peri-carditis	See Heart	
Peri-ostitis	See Bones	
Peritonitis	Also see Pelvic diseases	112
Pertussis (whooping cough)		113
Petechiae		113
Phthriasis (lice)		113

Petit mal epilepsy	See Epilepsy
Pharyngitis	113
Phlebitis (inflammation of veins)	113
Phlegmasia alba dolens (milk-leg)	113
Phobia (fears)	113,114
Phosphaturia	See Urine, sediments
Photophobia	114
Phthisis pulmonalis	See Tuberculosis
Pica (morbid appetite)	See Appetite
Pickles, excessive desire	See Appetite
Piles	See Hemorrhoids
Pityriasis (dermatitis exfoliativa)	114
Pleurisy	114
Pneumonia, broncho-pneumonia	114
Poisoning (decayed food)	115
Polio-myelitis	See Paralysis
Polychrome spectra, optical illusions	115
Polyps	115
Polyuria (copious urine output)	115
Portal congestion (also effective for piles)	116
Post-nasal diseases	116
Potatoes, disagree	See Appetite
Pregnancy, disorders	116,117,118
Pressure, ameliorates	See Amelioration
Priapism	See Chordee
Proctitis (inflammation of rectum)	118
Prolapsus, ani	118
Prolapsus, uteri (displacement)	118
Prolapsus, vaginae	118
Prosopalgia	See Neuralgia
Prostate gland	118
Pruritus, dermatitis, eczema	119
Psoriasis	119
Psychological disorders	See Moods 95

Pterygium	120
Ptosis	See Eyes
Ptyalism (salivation)	120
Pulmonary oedema (also see lungs)	120
Puerperium (lying-in period)	120
Pulse	121
Pupils	121
Purpura	121
Pyelitis (inflammation of pelvis of kidney)	121
Pyemia (pyogenic bacteria in blood)	122
Pylorus, diseases	122
Pyorrhoea, alveolaris	122
Pyrosis (heartburn) Also see Acidity, Dyspepsia	122
Pyuria (pus in urine)	122

R

Rectum	123
Reflux oesophagitis	26
Renal colic (also see kidney)	123
Respiratory paralysis	See Paralysis
Rest, ameliorates	See Amelioration
Retorbulbar neuritis with blindness	See Neuritis
Retina, diseases of	123
Rheumatism (Arthritis), joints, synovitis	124
Rhinitis (inflammation of nose)	124
Rickets	125
Riding. Aggravatges	See Aggravation
Ringworm (Trichophytosis)	125
Rising, aggravates	See Aggravation
Room, heated, aggravates	See Aggravation
Rubella (German Measles)	125

S

Salpingitis (inflammation of fallopian tubes)	126
Salt, excessive desire See Appetite	
Scabies(itch-mite)	126
Scalp, affections	126, 127
Sciatica	127
Scleroderma	127
Scleritis	127
Scrofulous diseases	128
Scrotum, eczema	128
Scurvy	128
Sea sickness, Travel Sickness	128
Sebaceous cyst	128
Seborrhoea (dandruff) See Scalp also	128
Sedentary habits See Aggravation	
Seminal vesiculitis	128
Seminal emissions See Emissions	
Senile decay (Aging)	128
Sensations	129
Septicemia (bacteria multiplying in blood), Also see Pyemia	129
Septicemia, Puerpural	129
Septum, ulceration, of nose	129
Sexual excesses, ill-effects of See Neurasthenia	
Shock See Adynamia	
Sinuses (Antrum, Sphenoid, Frontal)	129
Sitting, aggravates See Aggravation	
Skin diseases See Acne, Baker's itch, Barber's itch, Comedo, Ecchymoses, Frackles, Furuncles, Fungal infections, Leucoderma, Petechiae, Pityriasis, Pruritus, Psoriasis, Ringworm, Scalp, Warts.	
Sleeplesseness (insomnia)	130
Small-Pox (Variola)	130

Smell disorders	130
Smoking, aggravates	See Aggravations
Sneezing	130
Spermatic cords, affections (also see Neuralgia)	131
Spermatorrhoea and after-effects (see Impotence)	131
Sphinctres, paralysis	See Paralysis
Spinal cord	131
Spleen, affections	132
Sprains, strains	132
Spring, aggravates	See Aggravation
Squint	See Strabismus
Stage fright	132
Standing, aggravates	See Aggravation
Sterility (difficult or no conception)	132
Stomach, diseases	132
Stomatitis	132
Strabismus (Squint)	132
Straining, over-lifting, stretching	See Complaints
Strangury (difficult urination)	134
Summer heat, effects of	See Aggravation
Summer, ameliorates	See Amelioration
Sun, aggravates	See Aggravation
Surgical shock, anaesthetics	134
Sweat, disorders	134
Sweets, aggravate	See Aggravation
Sweets, excessive desire	See Appetite, perverted
Sycosis	See Barber's itch
Syncope (fainting)	135
Synovitis	135
Syphilis	135,136

T

Tabes dorsalis (Locomotor ataxia)	137

Tachycardia (rapid pulse)	See Pulse
Taenia (Tape-worm)	See Worms
Talking, aggravates	See Aggravation
Taste disorders	137
Tenesmus (See Strangury also)	137
Tea, excessive desire	See Appetite, perverted
Teeth, affections	138
Testes	139
Tetanus	140
Thirst	140
Thyroid gland	See Goitre
Tinnitus aurium (noise in ear)	140
Tobacco abuse	141
Tongue, diseases of	141, 142
Toothache	See Teeth
Tonsils	143
Tophi, gouty	See Nodosities
Touch, aggravates	See aggravation
Trachoma	See Eyes, granular lids
Trichophytosis	See Ringworm
Trigeminal neuralgia	See Neuralgia
Trismus (lockjaw, stiffness, tetanus)	143
Tuberculosis	143
Tumors	144
Typhoid fever	144, 145

U

Ulcers	146
Umbilicus	147
Uraemia	See Kindney diseases 147
Urethra	147, 148
Urinary diseases	148, 149

Urine, types	150
Urine, sediments	151
Urticaria (hives)	152
Uterus, diseases (also see Neuralgia)	152
Uterine polyps, fibroids	See Polyps

V

Vaccination, injection, ill-effects	154
Vagina, diseases of	154
Valvular diseases, of heart	154
Varicocele	155
Varicose ulcers	See Ulcers
Veins, affections of	155
Vertebrae, necrosis	101
Vertigo	155
Vision, disorders	156
Vital drains	See Aggravation-Causation
Vitreous opacities	156
Vocal cords, paralysis	See Paralysis
Voice, using (speakers, singers, teachers), aggravates	
Vomiting	157

W

Walking, child slow to learn	62
Warmth, ameliorates	See Amelioration
Warts (verruca)	158
Weakness, shock	See Adynamia
Weather, dry, ameliorates	See Amelioration
Whooping cough	See Pertussis

Women, Weakness	See Adynamia
Worm fever	158
Worm, intestinal	158
Wounds	159
Wrist, affections	159

www.ingramcontent.com/pod-product-compliance
Lightning Source LLC
Chambersburg PA
CBHW052347220526
45465CB00003BA/996